❖

DEEPENING THE
TREATMENT

❖   ❖   ❖

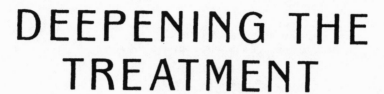

DEEPENING THE TREATMENT

Jane S. Hall, M.S.W.

A JASON ARONSON BOOK

ROWMAN & LITTLEFIELD PUBLISHERS, INC.
Lanham • Boulder • New York • Toronto • Plymouth, UK

Published by Jason Aronson
A wholly owned subsidiary of Rowman & Littlefield
4501 Forbes Boulevard, Suite 200, Lanham, Maryland 20706
www.rowman.com

10 Thornbury Road, Plymouth PL6 7PP, United Kingdom

British Library Cataloguing in Publication Information Available

Library of Congress Cataloging-in-Publication Data

The hardback edition of this book was previously cataloged by the Library of Congress as
follows:

Hall, Jane S.
  Deepening the treatment / by Jane S. Hall
    p. cm.
  ISBN 978-0-7657-0176-3
  1. Psychodynamic psychotherapy. 2. Psychoanalysis. 3. Psychotherapist and patient I.
Title.
  [DNLM: 1. Psychoanalytic Therapy. WM 460.6 H177d 1998]
  RC489.P72H34
  616.89'17—DC21
  DNLM/DLC
  for Library of Congress
  98-17723

ISBN 978-0-7657-0176-3 (cloth : alk. paper)
ISBN 978-0-7657-1009-3 (pbk. : alk. paper)
ISBN 978-1-4616-2812-5 (electronic)

♾™ The paper used in this publication meets the minimum requirements of American
National Standard for Information Sciences-Permanence of Paper for Printed Library
Materials, ANSI/NISO Z39.48-1992.

Printed in the United States of America

For Jim and Debbie

❖ ❖ ❖

Contents

✦ ✦ ✦

Acknowledgments

Doing psychotherapeutic work in private practice involves being alone with patients, day after day and year after year. As engrossing and rewarding as this is, it is also isolating. That is why my initial idea for this book was to invite a number of colleagues to join me. I like groups and a group effort seemed like a good idea. Also, it had never occurred to me to write a book. So when Jason Aronson said that based on my written proposal he liked my voice and asked if I would write the book myself I immediately answered no. "Think it over," he said. After a few days of spirited encouragement from my family and friends I agreed to try. My first thank you goes to Jason Aronson and the people who had faith in my ability to write down my ideas.

These ideas come from three sources: my patients, my students and colleagues, and my teachers. Martin Nass supervised me for ten years and his patience and wisdom saw me through difficult and often scary times. He taught me to view each patient as a unique person and never to fit a patient into a theory. He always said, "The patient writes the theory."

I was fortunate to be in a seminar with Gertrude Blanck for seven years after graduating from the Blancks' Institute for the Study of

Psychotherapy. The seminar had a core of students who, along with Trudy, made it a most stimulating learning environment. Her clinical expertise was awesome. Martin Bergmann, whom I first met while studying at the New York Freudian Society, was another inspiring teacher who taught me that there was something of value in every article and book we read and that even disagreement stretches our minds. As a member of his advanced seminar for many years I was privileged to learn from a true master.

I am greatly indebted to the people (colleagues, supervisees, and candidates) who permitted me to use their rich and inspiring clinical material. It has been a privilege to work with and learn from them and their patients. They are: Tom Afflerbach, Vivian Bader, Lauren Block, Louise Crandall, Linda Greenberg, Andrea Hadge, Paul Hymowitz, Christine Ranzoni, Susan Richenthal, Philida Rosnick, and Geraldine Wright.

As I began to see my words on the computer (I was completely computer illiterate until my daughter patiently taught me all I needed to know) I started to think I could write after all. That was before my good friend and colleague, Barbara Stimmel, agreed to take a look. Her talent always amazes me and her generosity in helping me improve the manuscript astounds me. I can't thank her enough.

Other colleagues and friends who gave me their valuable time, effort, and enthusiasm are Miriam Altman, Liz McKamy, Judith Mishne, Miriam Pierce, Arlene Kramer Richards, Arnie Richards, and Karen Trokan. They each had important comments and questions that gave me much to think about and to address. Their support and encouragement got me across the finish line. Joe Reppen's writing workshop reinforced my belief in avoiding jargon.

The Jason Aronson staff were gracious, supportive, and generous with their time. I thank particularly Cindy Hyden and Judy Cohen for their keen eyes and editorial expertise.

My daughter and my husband have both made important contributions to their fields. Without their inspiration, love, patience, and support I could not and would not have done this.

❖ ❖ ❖

Introduction: Perspectives

> If psychoanalysis survives into the next century, it will be because people at long last have come to value the imperishable truth that there is something to be said for being heard by an objectively neutral but empathically interested person who can withstand the rigors and bear the joys of an inner journey with a stranger.
>
> [James S. Grotstein 1994, p. 41]

Deepening the Treatment is based on the premise that almost everyone who crosses the therapist's threshold is looking for a second chance: a chance to live a richer, less restricted life. Second chances depend on the therapist's ability to show the patient that present life is colored by the past. Understanding how the echoes of the past resonate and shape one's life gives a person new choices and opportunities to resume development and resolve conflicts that are crippling. Such insight gives the patient a beginning sense of mastery not unlike the mastery achieved in learning a new skill.

It is up to us as therapists to see to it that our patients are presented with the "imperishable truth" of which Dr. Grotstein speaks. This book is meant to assist the psychoanalytically informed therapist in thinking about interpreting transference, countertransference, resistance, dreams, fantasies, and actions while helping her work in concert with the patient who will increasingly take over these interpreting functions. It will also consider how to help the patient recognize that this is a journey worth taking and that the therapist is a trustworthy guide.

Many people come to a therapist's office, whether in a clinic setting or in private practice, prepared to undertake weekly therapy (sometimes referred to as counseling). They often have little idea that their presenting problems are just the first few bars of their song. Weekly counseling is rarely enough to achieve lasting change but it is a reasonable way to begin. During the beginning stages the therapist has time to assess the patient's potential for psychological-mindedness, which is often overshadowed by initial anxiety. In this same period the patient has time to determine whether she feels enough rapport with the therapist to begin the gradual process of relating and revealing difficult, long-standing secrets. The way in which the therapist provides a safe environment while engaging the patient in psychoanalytic work, all the while maintaining her conviction that this work is effective in the face of the patient's despair and negativity, is the centerpiece of this book. All of this will rest on the task of gaining the patient's trust. The psychotherapist who respects the patient's pushes towards and pulls away from exploring her inner life is on the way to enabling the patient to trust in the psychoanalytic process.

This book is meant to help the beginning psychoanalyst who recognizes that analysis is the treatment of choice but is confronted by a patient who only wants counseling. It is for the clinician who knows that "fast cures" are rare and that, while short term therapy and behavior modification can help specific problems, they do not touch the deeper problems of living. It is meant to encourage the psychoanalytically oriented psychotherapist to consider training in psychoanalysis. Finally, it is for the mental health professional and the consumer interested in learning some of the basics of psychoanalytic technique.

This book considers psychoanalytically oriented psychotherapy to be on a continuum with psychoanalysis if the transference is recognized, respected, and worked with in contrast to the patient being advised and directed. Issues of frequency, fee, enactments, wishes to terminate prematurely, manifestations of transference, and the use of free association are discussed in terms of deepening the work and enlightening the patient.

The trials and the rigors of this work are as vast and difficult as they are rewarding. Like a guide who takes people mountain climbing, the psychoanalytically oriented therapist must have experienced both the dangers and pleasures of her own journey. Recognizing and working with the patient's transference inevitably leads to and involves the therapist's own transferences; her own personal psychoanalytic work allows the therapist to withstand and make use of these feelings.

Psychoanalytically oriented psychotherapy is an intensive form of treatment in which the therapist, maintaining a nonjudgmental attitude, provides a structure that permits the patient to explore her deepest feelings and fantasies. One of the greatest tests for patient and analyst repeatedly appears as the patient experiences the therapist as she once experienced early objects, often creating situations reminiscent of the past and of her unconscious fantasy world. The goal is to understand, both emotionally and intellectually, how and why the experiences and perceptions of the past affect the adult in the present. Throughout periods of reliving and reworking, a new perspective is gained so that development resumes, and the resolution of conflict and the ability to experience life through a new lens becomes possible.

Psychoanalytic work is surprisingly cost-effective. Like other forms of education, it has the potential to change one's life radically. Relationships deepen; work and professional goals become broader and realizable. Psychosomatic symptoms that are often very costly, sometimes involving years of medical bills, diminish and disappear.

Aside from those who come to my office either requesting or ready for psychoanalytic work, many of my patients have chosen to deepen the treatment as they come to understand how it works. People often need to wade rather than dive directly into deep water. It is for this reason that I wrote this book. Many patients begin therapy requesting direction and advice. The analytically informed therapist, with the goal of promoting autonomy, shows the patient that there are no fast answers, that advice would be a disservice, and that exploring ideas and expressing feelings are the most valuable tools leading to growth. It is the therapist's conviction in her work, her benign curiosity, and her skill that set the stage for deepening the treatment.

Chapter 1, "Setting the Stage," describes the psychoanalytic stance and discusses how the therapist provides a safe environment through her attitudes of respect and benign curiosity. Therapists who listen to patients with the idea that the presenting problems have roots in the past and are multidetermined have already deepened the treatment; listening is the key concept and technique. Many therapists, especially in the beginning, feel a pressure to relieve suffering before it is understood. Suggestions, advice, and other activity on the therapist's part usually serve to deprive the patient of the important opportunity to explore and to understand the problem.

"First Meetings," the subject of Chapter 2, are what determine the therapeutic dyad's decision to work together. When a prospective patient is seen by the therapist as an individual who has navigated life in the best way possible so far, the patient will feel less criticized and judged and more willing to look inside. How the therapist greets the patient in the first session, what she hopes to accomplish, and how she engages the patient in telling her story are the topics of this chapter. Efforts to diagnose, measure, and assess pathology must be counterbalanced by attitudes of respect and patience and with the spirit of inquiry and exploration.

"Deepening the Treatment," "Considering the Patient's Pace," and "Respecting the Patient and the Method," Chapters 3, 4, and 5, illustrate the concepts in previous chapters with case material from both clinic and private practice settings.

Chapter 6, "Separations between Patient and Therapist," deals with a subject that is crucial to understanding a most serious time in all treatment. I have presented some very basic issues such as how to prepare for a break and what to listen for to assist the therapist–patient dyad in deepening their work. Many patients threaten to end therapy before or after a planned break; separations, which so often cause painful anxiety, make these dangerous times in treatment. Case material illustrates how the anxiety is manifested, and how it can be understood and interpreted.

"Tolerating the Patient's Rage," the topic of Chapter 7, is very difficult for many therapists and yet very necessary to many patients. Hopefully, this chapter will make this often harrowing time more tolerable and understandable.

The last chapter, "From Psychotherapy to Psychoanalysis," is about swimming in the deepest waters. Psychoanalytic training that involves the therapist's personal analysis, intensive supervision, and course work is the only way to prepare for the undertow involved. This chapter describes and discusses the development of intense transference configurations and the difference between *working through* and *working out*.

The journey inward is arduous, fascinating, and rewarding. Time and money notwithstanding, there seems to be reluctance from both sides of the couch to make the journey. The myth that there is a paucity of "analytic cases" has frightened many psychotherapists who feel that analytic training is too expensive and that managed care is too formidable an obstacle to overcome.

For many years in this country psychoanalysis was presented as an elite medical specialty meant to treat only the "classic neurotic," and that is another reason that more analytic work is not being done. Times have changed. The climate, too, has changed. Traditional analytic institutes have opened their doors to nonmedical applicants. Other analytic institutes are now run by and train social workers, psychologists, nurses, and others. Private seminars and supervision are available so that formal institute training is not the only option.

Psychoanalytic work benefits people with all kinds of problems. It is now recognized that the most hard-to-reach patients are most in need of psychoanalytic treatment, the treatment that Wallerstein (1983) describes as, in many ways, the most supportive of all psychotherapies. Theoretical orthodoxy has been challenged, resulting in what is referred to as *theoretical pluralism*. A removal of certain strictures has invited the inclusion of interactive and interpersonal aspects of the analytic process not included in the traditional considerations of conflict interpretation. The analyst has evolved from a blank screen to a collaborator with functions and transferences of her own. A spirit of inquiry has replaced theoretical rigidity.

As we accept that psychotherapy can be deepened, we find that more and more patients are capable of engaging in this intensive form of treatment. Inflexibility has been a profound and pervasive criticism of analysts for the past fifty years. It used to be taught that psychotherapy interferes with establishing an analytic process. It was thought that psychotherapy involved techniques that preclude or make difficult the evolution of the transference neurosis. My experience shows the opposite. This book describes how to conduct psychotherapy in a way that deepens into the more intensive work of analysis when appropriate.

As stated earlier, psychotherapy, when conducted with analytic principles of theory and technique, is considered on a continuum with psychoanalysis. Once- or twice-weekly psychotherapy where transference phenomena are used by the therapist to aid the patient in understanding herself is a useful and effective form of psychoanalytic treatment. Not every adult patient is suited to analysis, especially in the beginning of treatment. I have seen patients move gradually into analysis, while some never do. Psychotherapy conducted twice a week is enormously helpful for some, while the more intensive work of analysis is more helpful for others. If we think in terms of deepening the treatment such dichotomies can be avoided. Those analysts who see psychotherapy as inferior to analysis miss out on moving and impressive work. Rothstein (1995) and his colleagues *"prefer doing analysis to psychotherapy . . . [and this way] the analyst thinking of himself doing analysis feels better about himself and his patient"* (pp. 5, 6). Bernstein (1983) and Levine (1985) take a moderate approach by conducting a phase of psychotherapy during which they show the patient her resistance and why she might fear deepening the work into psychoanalysis.

Deepening the Treatment is about establishing trust. A meaningful alliance with a therapist can take years of work. What sometimes seems like trust is actually compliance that must eventually be understood if real change is to occur. This is a slow process filled with tests for the therapist, particularly when a person has suffered real abuse in childhood or has been exposed to poorly conducted psychotherapeutic treatment.

Teaching courses on the theory of psychoanalytic technique for the past twenty years has, in turn, taught me a great deal. Watching candidates get turned on to the psychoanalytic concepts of neutrality, transference, resistance, the unconscious, psychic determinism, and interpretation continues to be gratifying and educational for me. Seeing therapists apply these psychoanalytic ideas to their work with patients is extremely rewarding to them, to the patients, and to me.

In this book I present many of the issues that have come up in my classes, in supervision, and in my own practice over the years. Questions such as how to respond to personal questions, how to respond to a patient's threat to end treatment prematurely, and what to do about requests for advice are among those issues that apply to a range of patients. The loudest question I hear has to do with how psychoanalytic techniques can be used with patients who do not come requesting psychoanalysis or psychoanalytically oriented psychotherapy and who sometimes know little if anything about psychoanalytic work. This book is my attempt to answer these questions.

My experience has led me to believe that psychoanalytic treatment is indicated when development has been derailed, when conflict has become inhibiting, and when there is a capacity for self-reflection. Assisting a prospective patient to be self-reflective will be discussed throughout this book. Our patients deserve the chance to continue developing, and psychoanalytic treatment often provides that chance. Believing this sincerely and profoundly allows us not to become bogged down with our patients' self-destructive values and ideas regarding time and money. Our kind of help is invaluable, unique, and necessary in affecting the quality of our patients' lives, and it is this confidence and belief in our work and our courage to do it that will be felt by our patients—because everyone wants a second chance.

❖ C H A P T E R   1 ❖

Setting the Stage— Providing the Structure (An Ongoing Process)

Psychoanalytically oriented psychotherapy is a journey inward. Travelers are always anxious to some degree. When the vehicle of transport seems safe and sturdy, and the pilot or captain impresses the passenger with her expertise and confidence, the traveler can relax to some extent. The therapist has the same obligation: providing a safe and secure environment for travel.

Many people who come to a therapist have felt betrayed early in life and therefore do not trust easily, if at all. Since the unique relationship between patient and therapist that evolves over time provides new opportunities for trusting, setting the stage is very important. The therapist's attitude of respect, patience, and benevolent curiosity combined with her confidence in the analytic process is what impresses the patient and permits her to stay in treatment. The persistent durability and constancy of the therapist and her functions presents the patient with a new reality, one that holds the potential for reviewing and experiencing the calamities of life in a new way. Differentiation becomes safe. Separations become bearable. Competition becomes acceptable. Feelings of effectiveness become more rewarding than feelings of omnipotence and grandiosity. Experiences of success and failure can exist side by side and do not cancel each other out. Closeness and intimacy become possible.

How do we set the stage for the deeper work that needs to be done? How do we create a safe environment? How do we pass the tests?

1. By having an inner conviction that each person has a unique story to tell, and respecting his or her way of relating it;
2. By listening carefully and following what the patient says attentively so that we can make connections and interpretations when appropriate;

3. By being confident that the long-term process of working through is necessary and possible for the patient to resume development and diminish conflict;
4. By being nonjudgmental, nonintrusive and open-minded;
5. By listening for strength as well as for pathology, and not letting premature diagnoses or diagnostic labels cloud the picture;
6. By being respectful of the patient's pace and autonomy;
7. By being firm and flexible when either are appropriate, and learning how to know when to be which;
8. By listening with respect, and by being comfortable not knowing the answers—or even the questions sometimes;
9. By encouraging and protecting the patient's curiosity and capacity for self-reflection;
10. By not burdening the patient with personal information and opinions;
11. By remembering that no two cases are alike, and that each patient creates her own theory (not fitting the patient into the theory);
12. By setting the conditions of treatment such as fee, payment, vacation policy, and missed session policy in the consultation phase so as to clear the way for work without distraction;
13. By remembering that *growth* and not *cure* is the goal;
14. By being consistent, reliable, calm, and benevolently curious;
15. By providing an atmosphere of trust, safety, and confidentiality.

Benevolent curiosity is a phrase I learned when reading Ella Sharpe's (1950) collected papers. Two chapters in this collection, "The Analyst," and "The Analysand," are basic reading for anyone who practices psychoanalytically oriented psychotherapy and psychoanalysis. Since psychoanalysis is a psychoanalytically oriented psychotherapy I will use the terms *psychoanalytic treatment* and *psychoanalytic work* most of the time. I reserve the term *analyst* for those clinicians who have undertaken their own personal analysis and analytic training. I use the term *therapist* to refer to all clinicians. I assign Sharpe's papers to every technique class I teach because they explain the essence of our work.

Sharpe says:

> The fundamental interest of a would-be technician must be in people's lives and thoughts. The dross of the infantile super-ego in that fundamental interest must by analysis be purged. The urgency to reform, to correct, to make different, motivates the task of a reformer or educator. The urgency to cure motivates the physician. *A deep-seated interest in people's lives and thoughts must in a psycho-analyst have been transformed into an insatiable curiosity which, while having its recognizable unconscious roots, is free in consciousness to range over every field of human experience and activity, free to recognize every unconscious impulse, with only one urgency, namely, a desire to know more and still more about the psychical mechanism involved. . . . When we come to a habit of thought, a type of experience, to which we reply: "I cannot understand how a person can think like that or behave like this," then we cease to be technicians. Curiosity has ceased to be benevolent.* [pp. 11, 12, italics added]

Benevolent curiosity comes easier to some than to others and is easier to practice with certain patients than others, but if we keep it as the most important stance to strive for we can interest the patient in deepening the treatment. One reason is that patients see therapists over time as nonjudgmental and worthy of their trust. Another reason is that through identifying with the analytic attitude patients become less critical and more curious. In fact, if there is one thing that engages patients in looking inside it is the ability to be benevolently curious about themselves. The therapist's spirit of inquiry is what makes analytic work possible.

Often, in the beginning of a treatment (and later on, too) the patient expresses curiosity about the therapist. This brings us to numbers 9 and 10: "not burdening the patient with personal information or opinions" and "encouraging the patient's curiosity and capacity for self-reflection."

Every therapist has heard different versions of the following words: "How can I have thoughts or feelings about you? I know nothing about you. If only I knew if you had children or were married or were ever divorced or used drugs or liked to cook or went to movies—then maybe I could trust that you'd understand me."

Beginning therapists often have difficulty not answering personal questions because they see this as depriving the patient and possibly damaging the alliance. In all my years of teaching, supervising, and treating I have found that once this therapeutic attitude of not answering questions is explained the patient feels safer and the treatment deepens. There are always exceptions to every guideline because each patient is unique and because different clinical situations require different responses. The stance of benevolent curiosity, however, usually saves the therapist from making uninformed decisions.

When a patient asks me a personal question I explain, with utmost tact, that questions are very important to the work of understanding but that by answering personal questions or giving personal opinions I would cut short an important learning opportunity. The opportunity is the patient's fantasy about the answer. I say something like, "Your questions are very important to me, and in a different setting it would be polite to answer. Here, we want to learn about your thoughts and feelings. Your questions about me are valuable ways to explore them. It would be easy for me to answer but in doing so I would be depriving you of a chance to wonder about and to picture me any way you want to." Such an explanation is basically reassuring to a patient. It says to her that there are boundaries; that this is not a social situation where politeness is required; and that her therapist is interested in helping her reflect. Said early in treatment it helps educate the patient about how the work is done.

How many of us have never answered a personal question? Therapists who do psychoanalytic work understand the idea of abstinence but because we learn best by experience most of us have answered a personal question or been tempted to offer advice. What we learn is that rather than help the patient trust, these answers often do the opposite. If the therapist answers one question, why would the patient not expect all questions, or at least most, to be answered? Answering questions takes away the patient's right to wonder and to explore her own fantasies. I have heard patients ask the questions and then reassure me that they really don't want me to answer. Despite the current debate on self-disclosure, with some analysts advocating the sharing of personal information and others preferring the traditional approach, it seems that if the therapist understands and respects the patient's right to imagine she will protect that right as best she can. There are some patients who cannot seem to tolerate a therapist's nondisclosing stance and it is at these times and with these patients that common sense and experience must guide us.

Telling a patient where you're going on vacation in most cases oversteps the bounds of the professional atmosphere so crucial to the work. It may seem like a minor point but if the analyst starts sharing personal information, how, when, and where does she draw the line? Telling a patient a little can be tantalizing, as if one says, "Take a peek, but only a peek." My preference is to give the patient the space to explore in fantasy where I go and to preserve my privacy. Of course, there are exceptions. A woman began therapy right before my winter vacation. In the last session before the vacation, when at the door, she said, "Oh, where are you going?" I asked if we could talk about it in a week when I returned. She never came back. I realized the minute this woman left that what I said had appeared rude. I had not yet had a chance to explain the value in exploring questions with this person. I have never made that mistake again. With most patients I respect their right to picture me wherever and with whomever they want. Thinking about the therapist as having a "real" life is difficult for some patients, especially toward the beginning of treatment. A patient who pictured me vacationing on an island with only books for pleasure gradually over the many years of work added a dog to the picture and eventually a family. Waterskiing replaced reading as issues of object loss, separation, envy, jealousy, and oedipal rivalry entered the treatment and were worked on. Taking away this patient's opportunity for fantasy by giving her facts would have deprived her of the chance to work at her own pace.

There are times when it is appropriate to tell a patient where you go on vacation. Someone who suffered from severe separation anxiety that seriously disrupted her functioning was able to maintain her stability by bringing an atlas to sessions prior to the vacation break.

Tracing the therapist's travel route was the patient's solution and the therapist respected this autonomous idea.

With a fragile patient who might be wounded rather than helped by not getting an answer the therapist might say something like, "I will answer your question but can you work with it first? This way we will learn more than if I answer you quickly. Then, if you still feel that my answering will be helpful, I will."

A different kind of challenge appears in the context of a bicycle accident I had many years ago while on vacation. When I resumed work my eye was black and I was still limping. I felt that my patients deserved an explanation so I told them the truth. One patient said, "Likely story! Your husband probably did it." This was said with a laugh but we were able to use her "joke" to tap into her anger at my absence and at my husband, whom she imagined as her rival for my attention. Some therapists might have chosen to wait for the patient's reactions. My self-disclosure in this case had roots in my unconscious. Any time the therapist makes a decision to disclose personal information it is most helpful if she analyzes her decision. The point is that there is no absolutely correct way for the therapist to be in the myriad situations that come up when working analytically, except to understand as best she can what motivates her and to preserve the frame whenever possible.

Mr. Baldwin asked in his first interview if the therapist was Catholic. He could not imagine how a non-Catholic could understand his background. The therapist said that although she understood his concern she was sure he could convey what it was like. Even if she was Catholic, that did not mean their experiences were identical. Her tone conveyed respect for his ability to articulate his experience and he was satisfied enough to continue treatment. The therapist could have explained in more detail the reason for her policy if the patient had persisted in knowing. She might have said something like, "It would be so easy for me just to answer your question but if I did it would deprive you of a chance to understand yourself on a deeper level by putting me in the spotlight instead of you. Our job here is to understand you. Sharing my experience would really not help us reach our goal of understanding." Such an explanation, when given respectfully, gives the patient more than the answer to the question asked. It gave Mr. Baldwin the message that the therapist believes in her method, is able to set a boundary, and is genuinely interested in exploring his fantasy and in valuing his curiosity. If the therapist had answered the question, Mr. Baldwin would have been deprived of picturing or imagining the therapist any way he needed or wanted to. Even a small bit of information can interfere with the patient's freedom to fantasize about the therapist.

A supervisee had to cancel her appointments in order to attend a funeral. She thought it would be polite to give the patients her reason so they would not think she was frivolous or unreliable. After discussing her rationale in supervision she realized that by giving this information she would curtail the patients' reactions to the cancellation. It is difficult to express anger and annoyance when a funeral is involved. Since a patient must feel free to express anger at the therapist she must be very careful about interfering with that ability. With very fragile patients the therapist must use clinical judgment. Our aim is not to harm a patient, it is to maintain enough anonymity to permit the development of transference fantasies. Personal information about the therapist becomes a burden because it usually requires a realistic response.

An action-prone, hostile patient responded to his therapist's last-minute cancellation with concern—the first nonsarcastic reaction in the treatment—by saying, "I hope everything is okay." Asked about his thoughts he said, "You're always here and always on time—something very important must have happened." This moment of reflection might have been precluded had a reason been given.

Being "always here and always on time" means reliability (number 14). Many patients have never experienced reliability, consistency, and respect. These three attitudes are required if the treatment is to deepen.

Even a commonplace question like "How are you?" becomes grist for the mill in psychoanalytic work. Mr. Spacey habitually greeted his therapist, Dr. P., with the same question. One day, Dr. P. pointed it out.

> *Therapist:* I notice that when I open the door you always ask how I am.
>
> *Patient:* Oh, it's just a habit—something I usually say.
>
> *Therapist:* I understand, but what are your thoughts?
>
> *Patient:* Well, I *have* wondered if you're tired. I must be your last patient of the day—I can't imagine how you concentrate.
>
> *Therapist:* What comes to mind?
>
> *Patient:* My wife is exhausted by the time I get home—the kids wear her out all day and we don't talk much in the evening. My mother was that way too. With all those kids none of us really got any individual time. [Mr. Spacey continues to reflect about his loneliness and eventually becomes aware of his anger and sadness at feeling neglected.]

It would have been easy for Dr. P. to let the "How are you" go because it is a socially accepted form of greeting. By approaching the question with benign curiosity he accomplished several things. He engaged the patient in looking beneath the surface, showing him that there were many feelings behind a simple, normal question.

Clinicians who are psychoanalytically oriented differ on the matter of how they address their patients (Fancher and Hall 1989). A question frequently asked by patients during a course of treatment, and often in the consultation phase is, "Will you call me by my first name?"

One of my first patients began seeing me in a clinic that specialized in drug-related problems. He was a charming, seductive homosexual who had been arrested for possession and for having a sexual encounter in a public men's room. The judge gave him a choice between jail and therapy. He chose the latter. After three appointments he asked if he could call me "Jane" so that he could relax and talk more easily about his drug use and lifestyle. He could also experience therapy as a friendly process instead of something he was required to do by the judge.

I agreed to his request because the agency therapists were almost all on a first-name basis with the patients, and I was concerned that by not granting his request I would injure him narcissistically.

What I want to point out with this seemingly understandable and well rationalized example is that granting this request without understanding its unconscious roots set a tone of avoidance that was hard to overcome in the many years of treatment that followed. Joe was a seriously disturbed man who was used to expressing his feelings through actions and dulling them through drug use. The treatment did deepen into analysis after several years of twice-a-week work, but there was always an undercurrent of teasing and refusing to take things seriously. I mention this case as an example of failing an early test that made later tests harder to pass. Looking back, I see that my countertransference was both induced and personal. It had to do with the seriousness of this patient's pathology, which he avoided seeing at all costs, and with my wish to be liked. This enactment was an unconscious collusion on both our parts to overlook the gravity of Joe's situation and the past that led to it.

Today, I would have dealt with that early test differently. I would say something like, "Your request is important and certainly understandable, but before we make any decisions can you try to explore your request some more?" I would go on to explain, if necessary, that if he allowed himself to see and say what came to mind we would be able to understand things in ways that would help us get to know him. I would say this with tact and sincerity but with a firm belief in my method. This way the patient would have a chance to learn about me, too. He would learn about my benevolent curiosity, my confidence in my method of working, and that he could not seduce me as he seduced everyone else in his life. He would also begin to see that reflecting about something is far more interesting and satisfying than acting first.

Using formal means of address usually makes it easier for the patient to express embarrassing material. First names imply a friendship to most people, and although the therapist is often experienced as a friend she is far more. The therapist is first and foremost a pro-

fessional. Second, and equally important, she is a transference figure. The formality of surnames serves as a frame for the transference
fantasies and feelings that will be expressed with time. I know from
my experience supervising that many therapists prefer using first
names. This is usually because their own therapy was conducted using
first names. Other reasons for using first names have to do with custom and culture. However the therapist decides to introduce herself,
it is important to understand a patient's request to change the form
of address once treatment has begun.

> After a year of analysis a patient told me that it had angered him when
> I referred to myself as Mrs. on his message tape when I returned his
> phone call. "Why can't I call you 'Jane'?" he asked. I asked him to talk
> about his anger and what it might mean to call me "Jane." After his
> associating to a distant mother I said that calling myself "Mrs. Hall"
> suggested to him that I was distant. I asked him to talk about that.
> Once the transference issue was addressed the name issue lost
> importance.

With a different patient I explained that she would be having all kinds
of feelings about me, would want to call me different names as the
treatment deepened, and that these feelings would be safe because
of the professional atmosphere of treatment. This was my way of
preparing her for transference. Like a guide telling a traveler some of
the things that might occur on a journey, I find it helpful to pave the
way with new patients by explaining that many different feelings will
come up.

Pressure to give advice is a dilemma for many therapists and I have
heard many examples of the therapist succumbing. Giving advice
often gets in the way of listening with benevolent curiosity. The
therapist's ability to engage the patient in exploring her conflict
around making a decision is ultimately what fosters the patient's
autonomy. Explaining this to a patient requires tact and timing, and
it is an excellent opportunity to increase the patient's own benevolent curiosity. Once the therapist makes the mistake of giving advice
it is difficult (but not impossible) to stop. There are many mistakes

we make, especially in the beginning. In supervision we learn new techniques and ways to hear things. There is nothing wrong in saying something like, "Although I have given you advice before, I think that by both of us looking at the question you will find a comfortable answer." Changing technique is not only permissible, it is necessary because we are always learning new and better ways to hear and respond.

The reasons to refrain from advising a patient are:

- Advice from a therapist is antithetical to the analytic work of understanding.
- Advice from the therapist assumes a value judgment.
- Advice infringes on a patient's autonomy.
- The therapist who gives advice is doing so often because of unanalyzed countertransference; there are so many ways to enlist a patient's decision-making skills without such advice.
- Once advice is given the patient may feel obligated to follow it.
- If the patient can't follow the therapist's advice, a whole new dynamic is introduced that can add to guilty or shameful feelings.
- If the patient does follow the therapist's advice and things go badly, it is more difficult to explore the meaning of what happened.
- There are usually plenty of people in a patient's life who offer advice. The therapist is usually the only one who cherishes the patient's ability to reach her own decision, for better and for worse.
- If a patient is about to make a destructive or damaging decision the therapist can always point that out and analyze why the patient is contemplating hurting herself.

It is important to understand with the patient why advice is requested. Understanding the request is far more useful in the long run than any advice the therapist might give. The demand or request for advice can be a test to see if the therapist can be consistent in her neutral, benevolently curious stance. Recently the concept of neutrality has been challenged by Stolorow (1990) and others (Panel

1997). I maintain that the analyst who takes a stand or makes a judgment one way or the other about most issues is stepping out of bounds. In most instances, taking sides interferes with the analyst's stance of benign curiosity and the patient's quest for autonomy. Examples in which a therapist might be tempted to make a value judgment include: whether a patient finishes or drops out of school, whether a patient considers giving up a seemingly important chance for professional advancement due to neurotic conflict, even whether the patient threatens to quit treatment. Taking a stand on such issues takes the therapist away from analyzing. For the analyst, the natural hope that a patient does the "best" or "right" thing must take a back seat to understanding why a patient chooses to do something. This is a test that happens in almost every case (especially in the beginning) and, if failed, can interfere with the patient's ability to trust. If a parental figure gives in to a child's demands frequently or randomly, the child will continue to test for boundaries. Love is behind the parent's ability to be consistent and firm. Rejection is expressed by a parent's inconsistent behavior. A therapist's ability to be firm and to set safe boundaries adds up to concern, something many of our so-called "difficult" or "borderline" patients have never felt sure of. For example, when a patient asks for advice about changing jobs or leaving home I say something like, "What's best for you is something only you can figure out. If you talk about it and see what comes to mind I think things will become clearer." If the patient persists in wanting me to take a stand I focus on the persistence by saying something like, "Let's try to figure out what's behind your wish for me to decide." If that fails to deepen the work I explain, "My giving advice would be presumptuous because I can't know what would be best. Can you explore the pros and cons of the different decisions available? That way we can learn more." When a patient is contemplating an action that clearly would put her in jeopardy I would say, "This choice will obviously result in pain (or loss, etc.). Why do you think you would take such a step?" If the patient has a pretty good idea what the best decision is and still needs the therapist's approval, I focus on that by saying something like, "My approval seems so important to you. Can you talk about that?"

Mr. North sought treatment because he was depressed. The analyst he was referred to chose to help the patient assert himself by giving advice and encouragement. The analyst recommended books to read and plays to see. Mr. North was reminded of a Mel Brooks/Carl Reiner comedy record in which the analyst says to a patient whose problem is "tearing paper," "Don't tear paper." Mr. North realized that advice such as this was not what he was paying for and left treatment. Had the analyst interested Mr. North in why he had difficulty in asserting himself, he might have stayed in treatment.

Striving for a neutral stance does not mean that the therapist is a blank screen or mirror. Indifference is not what we feel or wish to convey. When a therapist hears that a patient is setting herself up for mistreatment or abuse she says something like, "It sounds like you're asking for trouble to me. Can you talk about that?" If the patient is behaving in a way that threatens a relationship or a job this must be pointed out with concern by the therapist, but advising or directing is not an analytic technique.

Feeling neutral when hearing about mistreatment is impossible and it is not unusual for the therapist to feel angry with her patient's abuser and with the patient for letting herself be abused or for abusing others. Expressing outrage and pain, however, is the patient's right, and assisting her to exercise that right is the therapist's goal. If the therapist actively takes sides she risks soothing the patient before the intense feelings that have often been avoided for years surface in the transference.

An exception to the guideline of not taking a stand involves a patient's suicidal behavior or threats. In such cases the therapist's first concern is the patient's health and safety. Involving the patient's family or friends and recommending hospitalization when appropriate are measures the therapist takes.

The stance of benign or benevolent curiosity is really the foundation of psychoanalytic work. If the therapist is consistent about this attitude the treatment will deepen naturally. Consistency and constancy apply to all the therapist's policies and to her demeanor. Being ready for the patient is important, even when the patient is late. While I do not feel that reviewing the previous session notes is usually necessary, I do try to clear my mind of distractions and to be aware of my feelings about seeing the patient.

A supervisee once had to move her office twice within one year. Her patients had varying reactions from annoyance to anger to fear. The disruption affected some more than others. A patient who had moved often during childhood was particularly upset. It took her time to adjust and she gained new understanding about just how upsetting her childhood moves were. New material emerged and was useful in understanding her need for consistency and her need for control.

One day she was late and found her therapist working at her desk when she arrived instead of sitting in her chair as she usually was. She became angry and talked about her fear of interrupting her therapist doing something she shouldn't see. This led to primal scene material heretofore repressed or avoided.

Although this material was useful I believe that it is important to be sitting in your chair, ready for the patient when she is late. I do not talk on the phone while waiting in case the patient is trying to call. It is important to convey to the patient that you are ready during her time.

I learned early in my training that there are two things you can guarantee a patient: the first is consistency and being on time is part of that; the second is your undivided attention. This means not taking phone calls during a session. It also means not drinking coffee during sessions. I have heard of therapists who work early in the morning and have coffee while the patient is on the couch. This seems disrespectful, impolite, and distracting to me. This also holds true when the patient brings coffee. I find eating and drinking during a session distracting and probably symbolic of something I don't understand. When a patient brings food or drink I say with all the tact I can muster something like, "Can we explore what bringing coffee to your session might mean?" If the patient takes this request as a rejection or seems angry I ask her to express these feelings. I then say calmly and tactfully something like, "I have found that eating and drinking

during the session can be distracting and can interfere with our work."
If the patient seems hurt or angry I ask her to tell me what she is
feeling. With a fragile patient I might add that my request is not meant
to deprive but to make our work easier.

Many therapists say that the patients they call *borderline* cannot
tolerate the abstinence required in analysis. (The word *difficult* has
replaced the term *borderline* with many therapists. This is a step away
from labeling but *difficult* describes the therapist's problem. I prefer
the word *troubled* or the phrases *deeply troubled, self-destructive, lacking in the capacity to self-regulate or self-soothe, fragile,* or *disturbed*
because they are more descriptive and less judgmental.) These therapists advocate parameters such as giving advice, answering personal
questions, not charging for missed sessions, and so on. I have found
that patients respond best to explanations for different analytic policies and poorly to parameters that they find infantilizing and patron-
izing. If the therapist can convey her respect and confidence in analytic work the patient will feel respected and more convinced about
the analytic process. Most of all, the patient will see that the therapist is not frightened of expressions of anger and disappointment.

These guidelines are meant to ensure consistency and to show respect. Naturally, because we are human, we will be late at times, and
if there is an emergency in our lives we may have to answer the phone.
If a patient is having an anxiety attack or is in emotional upheaval I
don't bring up the coffee issue at that time. Common sense is our
most valuable asset.

There are times when a patient may be seriously considering taking an action that is self-injurious, such as marrying someone who
seems dangerously inappropriate or quitting a job that would compromise her self-sufficiency. One patient was planning to tell off her
boss in a hostile and impulsive manner, thereby jeopardizing her job.
If poor judgment is being exercised the therapist can ask the patient
to talk about the pros and cons of her intended action. Aside from
suicidal or dangerous actions, however, it is risky to take a definite
stand. The risk lies in shifting from the neutral, benevolently curious
attitude we strive for.

Ms. Weston was furious at her boss and had written a letter of resignation that she was about to mail. The boss indeed sounded like a difficult person but I wondered to Ms. Weston if there was anything else that had exacerbated her anger recently. She told of a conversation with her older sister who indeed reminded her in ways of the boss. I wondered if she felt that it was worth losing a good job to punish the boss who in many ways stood for someone else. Her rage did not subside immediately but thinking about things from a different angle bought her some time. When she cooled down she modified her strategy and asked for a transfer at work. This anger at the boss had reached a crescendo a week after I announced my summer vacation date. I asked Ms. Weston if she had some feelings and thoughts about my announcement. She began to see that she resented my calling the shots and saw that this reminded her of the boss and her sister, who always seemed to have special privileges. Ms. Weston had only been in treatment for six months and this was our first opportunity to hear about her feelings towards me. These feelings are known as *transference manifestations* (see Chapter 3). In the following session Ms. Weston brought up the boss's unfairness again and I asked if she thought my vacation felt unfair on some level. "Well," she said, "it did seem unfair that just as things were getting interesting you would decide to take a vacation." We learned that Ms. Weston's wish to get rid of or leave her boss was connected to my getting rid of her. If she could leave first, the pain of being left could be avoided. Using Ms. Weston's material to focus on her feelings about me set the stage for further work in the transference.

Mrs. Jenkins tested me from day one. She was always flirting with danger and had been for most of her life. She described a childhood of emotional abuse. A rejecting mother tethered her to a tree when she was 2 and 3 because she wandered away from home. We wondered if even at that age she was trying to get away or to seek something better. At age 8 she was left in charge of a younger cousin who ran out into the street where she saw him hit by a car. These facts combined with others led to guilt and rage that were usually self-directed. Mrs. Jenkins said she owned a gun for protection on an isolated farm in the country and threatened to take it on vacation. I did as much interpreting of her feelings about our separation as I possibly could and finally told her that, although I had no power to keep her from taking or even owning a gun, I certainly thought it was a very dangerous thing to do. The difference between advising Mrs. Jenkins not to take a gun and sharing my thoughts about it is a subtle one. You might say I offered my perception strongly but left the decision up to her. When Mrs. Jenkins returned from vacation and we resumed our work she told me that she had gotten rid of the gun and had really meant to frighten me. It was important that I did not try to force her to give up the gun and also that I showed my concern.

Before a vacation break Mr. Farnon told his therapist that he took LSD or amphetamines on occasion. He was an unstable and frightening patient in many ways but showing fear would have frightened him away. The therapist could only express concern. Before the vacation the therapist mentioned that if things were getting out of control Mr. Farnon could go to his hospital emergency room for help. The therapist suggested that he visit his local hospital so he knew exactly where to go. He was also given the name of a covering therapist to call if he wished. Again, expressing concern while allowing the patient to be responsible for himself proved very meaningful to this very disturbed young man.

A patient once told me that had I become involved in his life outside of the office he would not have continued treatment. He needed to rely on my ability to help him question his life and behavior, not to direct him. He had people to call in emergencies and his family was always advising and telling him what to do.

Every therapist gets drawn into action at times. A supervisee told me about a patient whose husband was exhibiting severe manic-depressive symptoms. My supervisee acquiesced to her patient's request to speak with her husband's psychiatrist, who seemed not to realize the severity of the husband's depression. The supervisee felt pulled into the marital problems and out of her inquiring stance. This supportive activity is required at times. Later on, when the outside or reality issues settled down, the supervisee and her patient were able to focus on the patient's internal life and her reactions to the therapist's involvement. Speaking to a third party on a patient's behalf is not recommended unless a situation reaches crisis proportions. When the therapist does intervene, it is important to obtain written permission. In most cases the patient should be present or should see the communication.

The structure, frame, and therapeutic environment are supportive in themselves. A patient once said, "When I come here I know you won't react each time I present a dilemma. You give me time to gain my perspective—to look at things from different angles. It's such a relief to have time to think things through. My friends and family are always putting their two cents in—giving me advice or cautioning me. When I started therapy I remember asking you for your opinion and for advice. It took me a while to realize that you respected my ability to think about things and come up with my own answers. And even if I goofed I would learn something."

There are two major sources of confidence (number 2). Our own analyses provide a model and convince us that the unconscious is both powerful and decipherable. Our work with our own patients substantiates these findings. When this confidence flags I have found that supervision or consultation is enormously helpful. Another source of confidence building is, of course, our studies. Even after formal training, study groups keep us in touch with psychoanalytic concepts and case material. After many years of analytic work with a man who seemed unable to alter his sadomasochistic life style and character structure both patient and analyst felt they had reached a stalemate. The analyst's countertransference began compromising her ability to be benevolently curious. Instead she felt that her own sadism, mixed with disappointment and frustration, was causing her to interpret in an impatient tone of voice. Such enactments are not unusual and can actually deepen the work if analyzed, but they are not always easily and satisfactorily analyzable. After consulting a supervisor for a period of time and returning to the literature on this subject she was able to regain her confidence. The articles brought her new understanding and made her feel less alone with her patient, who was pushing her away and trying to kill her effectiveness. Reading and consulting allow us to see that we are not alone.

Listening with respect and being comfortable not knowing the answers or even the questions (number 8) involves the technique of silence. If the therapist thinks about silence as active listening it is often easier to practice. The therapist's silent stance is not withholding, it is quite the opposite. How many patients have felt listened to in a nonjudgmental, attentive way before therapy?

Sometimes a patient begins therapy saying, "I don't want a silent therapist. I need you to talk and not just sit there." The therapist's response to this kind of statement can be used to educate the patient about the method of work. I usually say something like, "Listening to you is the best way I have of getting to know you. I promise you that when I think of something to say I will say it, but in the beginning it is especially important for me to hear you. When I am quiet I am concentrating on what you're saying." The patient may then continue to need assurance that you are paying attention, but your facial expression and an occasional question in face-to-face treatment usually allays that anxiety. Once the patient begins using the couch she is used to her therapist's listening stance. Some patients become anxious when they cannot see the therapist's face but a few words of reassurance usually suffice. If there is history of loss or neglect a deeper interpretation can often be made connecting the patient's present reaction to the past. This in itself encourages the patient's curiosity and ability to reflect. It also is a way to introduce the concept of transference.

When treating a patient who grew up with parents who rarely spoke the therapist will not want to repeat the experience by extreme silences, but even in such cases there are ways to be more actively quiet. "Hmm," "I see," "Can you tell me more about that?" "Is that a familiar feeling?" assure the patient that you are actively listening and present. The psychologist Carl Rogers had a way of repeating or echoing what the patient was saying, and this is another technique to consider when the patient is afraid or anxious about the therapist's silent stance.

The therapist's ability to be silent is extremely important in analytic work. Only when the therapist stays out of the way can the patient feel free to follow her thoughts without interruption. When a patient is given the opportunity to see where her thoughts go the idea of free association becomes sensible, reasonable, and informative. All the therapist has to say when the patient complains that there is nothing to say is something like, "See what comes to mind." If more explanation seems necessary the therapist can say something like, "It will help us understand things if you can see where your thoughts lead. If I talk a lot my words and thoughts will get in your way." This approach seems more sensible to me than talking about a "fundamental rule." Appealing to a patient's sense of logic enlists the patient's ego. Giving a rule invites a power struggle or a compliant attitude.

Saying what comes to mind can feel threatening to a patient and she may need encouragement. When this is the case the therapist can say something like, "Something *always* comes to mind. If you find yourself editing or withholding a thought you can try to figure out why. If you're afraid of saying something that seems embarrassing or if you're afraid of my reaction we can try to understand why." When a patient says, "My mind has gone blank," the therapist can say, "This often means that there are thoughts about me going on."

I find nothing wrong in explaining to a patient in the beginning of treatment that analytic work is done by seeing where thoughts lead (free association). I also say something like, "You'll be having thoughts and feelings about me as we go along and it will be helpful if you talk about them along with whatever else comes to mind." This approach differs somewhat from the stereotyped approach in which the analyst points to the couch after the first session and waits.

Since the majority of our patients do not come to us asking for analysis or even to do psychoanalytic work, it is up to the therapist to present her method of work in a way that makes sense. Patients are consumers and have a right to know something about the journey that they contemplate taking. This approach falls under the heading of respecting the patient and having confidence that saying what comes to mind and expressing feelings is valuable and leads to understanding.

Some therapists go to the other extreme, perhaps in reaction to a rigid approach. I have heard of therapists who invite patients to their homes or who have lengthy phone conversations as friends would.

Their rationale is that they are providing an experience they feel the patient missed in childhood or adolescence. I once heard of a therapist giving his patient a picture of himself before a vacation to "promote object constancy." Another therapist gave her patient recipes because the patient was a newlywed and felt she could not cook for her husband. These actions are not psychoanalytic techniques and must be considered supportive therapy at best. Such techniques and others like them overstep professional bounds and threaten the safe environment necessary to analytic understanding. They are usually the beginning of the end of treatment. The therapist's consistency, benign curiosity, and respect for a patient's autonomy are more supportive than the more active techniques just mentioned. With very anxious and fragile patients phone contact between sessions is sometimes necessary, but I have found that brief conversations are usually enough. The wish to talk between sessions can be a clue that more frequent sessions are appropriate. I have supervised a number of cases where the patient picks up on the therapist's anxiety and feels the need for contact between sessions. Once the therapist deals with her own anxiety either in her own treatment or in supervision the patient calms down.

The psychoanalytically oriented therapist will work towards promoting autonomy even in the most fragile patient. I have known patients who hold onto a bill or call the therapist's tape to hear her voice during vacations. The patient uses creative and autonomous ways of enhancing object constancy. This corresponds to the infant's choice of the transitional object. The mother cannot influence that choice.

Knowing when to be firm and when to be flexible (number 7) is a complex issue. Our firmness is extremely important to the patient who is testing our strength and conviction. Many therapists use their wish to be courteous, to be liked, and to form an alliance as reasons to alter their technique or to disregard the frame. A common example is letting the session go over. This is usually a mistake because it threatens the stability and safety of the hour. I have treated many patients who present a dream or other important-sounding material or affect in the last few minutes of a session. They often do this because it is anxiety-provoking and they feel safer knowing that the hour is almost up. If we go overtime the patient loses the safety net she consciously or unconsciously set up. In these situations it is important to stick to the boundary of the session. At such times there are different things we might say to the patient such as:

"I think if you start here next time we will learn something, but we must stop for today."

"This dream can tell us a lot, and your leaving it to the end also tells us something."

"It sounds as if you need more time. Once a week makes it difficult to get everything in. We could talk about adding another session next time" (see Chapter 3).

Comments like these respect the patient's pace while acknowledging her timing. As with all guidelines there are exceptions. When a patient is expressing intense affect towards the end of an hour the therapist wants to help her regain her equilibrium. I will say something like, "Our time will be up soon. I know you are very upset but for today can you calm yourself? Your feelings are so important to us but we must stop in a few minutes." These comments or others like them are said in a calm, respectful, concerned way. They are meant to assist the patient in composing herself and let her see that feelings do not have to be overwhelming to either party. If we allow extreme emotionality to go unchecked at the end of a session we may frighten the patient, and her trust in our knowing what's best is compromised.

Here the test involves the therapist's ability to be in charge and to protect the patient. It also has to do with the therapist's ability to provide structure and not to be seduced into changing it. There are patients who find it very difficult to leave and who linger. When this happens I recommend walking to the door and if necessary opening it to let the patient see that the time is indeed up.

Another test involving reliability and consistency is the request for changes in appointment times. Again, the ability to know when to be firm and when to be flexible comes into play. I have found that every request for a change must be explored first. If the request is well founded, and if I can reschedule, I will. However, it is important to listen for a reaction about the change in time. Patients come to rely on a permanent schedule and any shift can evoke memories of impermanence and inconsistency. Many patients have histories of unavailable caretakers and insecure early environments. This is why the therapist's consistency is so important. Experience teaches us that a secure frame is required for in-depth work. Accommodating a patient may seem polite but is often a way to say "Don't be angry."

One patient said she was getting to work late and asked if she could be seen at 7:55 AM instead of at 8:00. The therapist, not wanting her patient to get in trouble, agreed to the request without exploring it. The patient accepted the new time but instead of appreciating her therapist's flexibility she felt uncomfortable in getting her way so easily. This reaction allowed the issue of trust to be explored. It emerged that the patient feared being able to seduce the analyst into giving her what she wanted.

It is important and easier for both therapist and patient to stick to a schedule. A policy of shifting appointments for either party makes a steady pace of work difficult. Needless to say, rigidity is not the goal—stability is.

Patients try in many ways to seduce us. It is not that they come in one day with a plan to get us to shift our stance or change a rule. It is usually a more unconscious process and it is really a very reasonable way for the patient to determine just how professional and strong we are. The patient is seeking professional help, not friendship, when she chooses a therapist.

A colleague's patient asked for a progress report after two months of analysis. It was clear to the analyst that the patient was anxious about going deeper. The patient was a lawyer who was the head of his law firm, and progress reports were part of his life. The analyst felt intimidated at first but after some reflection told the patient that progress reports were not part of analytic treatment and wondered if there were feelings behind the question. This answer let the patient see that the analyst knew what was best and opened the door for the expression of feelings. The patient had been testing the analyst's strength and was relieved not to have frightened the analyst into answering. This patient had cut down his hours once before and he was re-testing his analyst's conviction and confidence in his method.

A difficult situation for some therapists is a patient's invitation to attend a concert, marriage, art show, or some other very important event. Some therapists accept such invitations, but I have found that exploring the request or invitation like any other question is the first order of business. Usually after the request is explored and it is understood what the effect on treatment would be, saying no is not necessary because the patient realizes that the therapeutic relationship would be compromised. With some patients, however, a courteous explanation about the therapist's reason for declining the invitation is necessary and welcomed by the patient in the long run.

A candidate told about a patient who in the first session asked her to see his art exhibition at a local gallery because he felt that this would help the therapist understand him. While at the gallery (the patient was not present) the therapist read the guest book. In it she noticed a lovely comment from the patient's mother. The patient had complained about his cold, disapproving mother and seeing the comment made the therapist question her patient's perception of the mother.

This is a good example of why we try to stay in the office. We owe our patients neutral listening. If a patient tells us something that makes us wonder about their perception this is appropriate because we are listeners with investigative ears, but hearing or seeing information from anyone but the patient compromises our ability to hear with objectivity. Complete objectivity is impossible to achieve for many reasons but it is something we strive for. (This is why it is best not to share information with a therapist who treats a friend or family member of your patient.) If the therapist remembers that she is being hired by the patient she will find it easier to listen only to the patient.

> During the termination phase of a long psychoanalysis, a patient invited his analyst to his wedding. It was a milestone in his life that he wanted her to share. The analyst was very moved and pleased at his success but declined the invitation. As much as she would have liked to attend she knew that her presence would be inappropriate on several levels. First of all, the patient had known her in a professional atmosphere for fifteen years. The special relationship they had developed with all of its ups and downs, love and hate, frustration and reward was unique and had to remain private. Overstepping the boundaries of this relationship would have made it vulnerable. They had not yet terminated and, even if they had, seeing each other outside of the office would have compromised the analytic atmosphere.

This may seem like a rigid or strict approach to some therapists but most patients are relieved by this therapeutic stance. Patients understand that extra-analytic meetings can threaten their work. Also, once a therapist ceases to protect the frame with one patient, she will be worrying about when, why, and if to do so with another patient. Having to make such decisions is stressful and takes us away from our analytic work. We begin to make value judgments and decisions that distract us from our purpose. Preserving the analytic atmosphere is our most important function and, although I realize that analysts do make exceptions, I have found that passing the test of consistency is one of the most important.

Training analysts differ about the need to avoid extra-analytic contact when analyzing a candidate. When the patient belongs to or is in training at the same institute it can be difficult to avoid such meetings. Some analysts believe that during the analysis of a candidate the candidate should have the choice of attending an analytic function and the analyst in such cases should defer. There are other ways to handle this kind of situation. For example, patient and analyst can discuss the situation and agree on what to do, having analyzed it first.

The main idea is to analyze the issue. The fantasies that are stirred up by seeing the analyst with other people in other settings are myriad and naturally become grist for the mill.

Charging for missed sessions is another problem for many of the people I have taught and supervised. The rationale can be traced to Freud, who conceived of treatment as leasing his hours. Practically speaking, the therapist is a professional person earning a living. If a patient cannot keep one or some of her appointments the therapist should not be penalized. Electricity, rent, and other bills continue whether our patients are there or not. If all or half of our patients cancelled in a given week the financial loss would be great. Having a policy that includes all patients is one way of avoiding favoritism or unequal treatment. The fact that we protect ourselves by charging for missed sessions may upset a patient initially, but this policy has never lost me a patient. To the contrary, patients feel safer when they see that therapists can take care of themselves. As for rescheduling appointments, that is an individual decision. Some therapists have the time flexibility and can change their schedules. I recommend that if rescheduling is possible, it be done in the week of the missed session. A request to reschedule can have many meanings, conscious and unconscious. The therapist who acquiesces quickly and frequently may be saying, "Don't be angry, see how accommodating I am." I learned an important lesson early on. I found that when I rescheduled an appointment without fully understanding the patient's request I would sometimes forget the new time. I learned that I found shifting appointments distracting to the rhythm of my work. I also found that often a patient would be upset with a new time and would forget to come or would resent my flexibility.

There are different ways of explaining this policy of paying for missed sessions. For a patient who has a job with sick day and vacation benefits, it is fairly easy just to state the policy. For people who travel regularly for work something more flexible can be arranged. Some therapists hold the missed time but charge half the fee; others make up the time. This is most difficult when the patient is in analysis because of the frequency of sessions. Whatever the policy, being firm is part of being consistent. It also conveys to the patient that we can tolerate anger. This is a major test that must be passed continually if the treatment is to deepen.

I have heard of patients who ask why they are not paid when the therapist is away. This is not a logical question and must be explored. All of these discussions are best done in the beginning of treatment. Towards the end of the first session or consultation phase when times are being arranged I say something like, "We will meet on Tuesday and Thursday at 6 PM. These times are yours. They belong to you and if for any reason you can't be here you will be responsible for them." I have had a patient cite a friend's therapist who does not charge if there is 24-hour notice. I said something like, "I imagine different people have different ways of working but I have found this works best for me."

This policy also entails being paid on time. Being a psychotherapist is difficult and serious work. Training and supervision, conferences, and reading are necessary and time-consuming. Being paid as well as you can be is important. The psychotherapist is not a philanthropist or a banker who extends credit. If a patient tries to build up a debt with us it is inappropriate. Borrowing money from a relative, friend, or bank or putting off treatment until one can pay protects the safety of the analytic atmosphere (see Blanck and Blanck 1974). Maintaining our professional identity is extremely important for us and for our patients.

I can usually think of an exception to any guideline but it is difficult with this one. It is only when we respect and take care of ourselves that we can do the same for our patients. No matter how kind and generous we are, we do a disservice by extending credit. If a patient loses a job or her source of income, we can decide to lower the fee or even to waive the fee (if absolutely necessary) temporarily. I recently heard that some analysts, because of managed care, arrange to have the patient pay them for uninsured sessions after the analysis is completed. I don't have enough information about how this policy works or how it affects the work so it would be wrong to comment at this time. Needless to say it is a policy that must have different meanings for different patients and would have to be analyzed in all cases.

Mrs. Cohen worked twice a week in psychotherapy for four years. During this time she was able to extricate herself from a destructive marriage, and began seeing what led her into it in the first place. Her ability for self-reflection, for reporting dreams and associating to them, and for exploring her feelings about me was evident. Due to her changed financial situation after the divorce she could no longer afford twice-a-week sessions even at a very reduced fee. I felt that analysis would greatly benefit Mrs. Cohen and I explained why. After a six-month period of work she chose to accept a referral to an analyst who would see her for a very low fee, making it possible for her to have the treatment of choice. Her original problem had been dramatic, and a long period of work on separation issues alleviated her anxiety to the point where she could function independently. She also had time to test the constancy and consistency of the therapist and to see that looking inside made sense and was helpful. Psychoanalysis had not been the initial treatment of choice for Mrs. Cohen but it became so, and when it did she was helped to pursue it.

Had Mrs. Cohen been able to continue her twice-a-week sessions at the original fee I still would have recommended analysis because that had become the treatment of choice. If I had been in the early phase of my practice with the time and need for an analytic case I would have discussed reducing Mrs. Cohen's fee and deepened the work into analysis myself. The psychotherapy we had done did not include measures that would have contaminated the transference. In this case my reality and her need made it a clear-cut issue. Unfortunately there are therapists who prefer to hold on to a patient at once or twice a week rather than refer to an affordable analyst. They rationalize that they are more experienced than a beginning analyst is and that the patient will be in better hands with them. I question this assumption. Beginning analysts are in excellent supervision and furthermore the frequency of analysis makes it easier for the patient to tolerate the anxiety inherent in deepening the work.

In Mrs. Cohen's case diagnosis was not an issue in my mind. I saw no need to give her a label at any time during treatment (see Chapter 2). When she came to treatment her separation issues and her masochism stood out. Her anger at her husband was turned against herself. During the four years we worked together she gradually felt safe enough to direct her anger towards me and she learned that I could not be destroyed by it. Her dependency needs manifested themselves in a perverse symptom. It became clear that analysis would be required to effectively deal with her issues. One well-known psychoanalytic institute rejected her for analysis based on a borderline diagnosis. An equally reputable one accepted her. I share this information to remind us of number 5. A person's resilience, psychological-mindedness, and motivation are far more meaningful than a diagnostic category. Mrs. Cohen is evidence that respecting the patient's pace and permitting the treatment to deepen by passing the tests on both sides of the couch lead to growth. The stage had been set for Mrs. Cohen's growth and she responded quite naturally.

When and how does the therapist raise her fee? This is a question often asked and discussed. There is a school of thought that once a patient decides to undertake analysis the therapist is bound by the original fee. I find this impractical and unrealistic. There are several issues to consider:

1. *Inflation:* some therapists raise their fees every year.
2. *Countertransference:* after a number of years of hard work the therapist can begin to resent not having a raise just like any other employee.
3. *Higher income:* the patient's ability to earn more money as a result of therapy warrants an increase in fee if the patient began at a reduced fee.

I find it easiest to raise the fee in January. I announce the fee raise in November when I give my bill to the patient. This advance notice gives the patient time to respond. Some therapists say to the patient before the August break that the fee will be raised in September. I find that with all of the feelings about vacation this is not the best time to bring up the fee. When a patient becomes able to pay more than the original fee, especially if the fee was a reduced one, it often appears in the material, either directly or indirectly.

To sum up, two people who decide to work together in psycho-analytic psychotherapy must both be as comfortable as possible. It is the therapist's responsibility to create a safe environment for the patient and a workable environment for herself. The therapist must consider her needs according to where she is in her personal and professional life just as she considers her patient's needs.

Therapists who practice psychoanalytic psychotherapy become more adept at deepening the treatment as their own analyses deepen. Only by recognizing and analyzing our own conflicts can we deeply appreciate and empathize with the conflicts of our patients. We must be able to look inside ourselves in an intensive and extensive way before we can guide another on the journey of self-exploration. Our own analyses prepare us for the rigors of our work and give us proper and deep respect for the unconscious. Our own analyses prepare us for the intense, often uncomfortable transferences and projections we must endure, understand, and interpret. Our own analyses enable us to recognize and deal with the induced and personal countertransference we are bound to experience. We are the recipients of all sorts of projections and feelings and our own analyses give us the courage and stamina to endure them.

All of these abilities are conveyed from unconscious to unconscious—the way most important information travels. Our insecurities, fears, and weaknesses, though ever present to some degree, can be sufficiently mastered, allowing us to set the stage for deeper work.

CHAPTER 2

First Meetings—
The Consultation Phase

Many people experience the decision to see a therapist as difficult, and making and keeping the first appointment is a major step. Sometimes the pressures and pain one experiences make the decision to start easier, but after a period of therapy, when symptoms abate and pain diminishes, the patient often wants to stop. If the original problem was minor, ending the treatment after specific goals are accomplished is usually appropriate. However, when the psychoanalytically oriented therapist determines that the symptoms and psychic pain have deep roots that must be tended in order for lasting change to occur, she is ethically bound to inform the patient that deeper, long-term work is the treatment of choice. Showing this to a patient requires skill, tact, and knowledge. The therapist's confidence in and conviction about the psychoanalytic process and her ability to convey this is a major determinant in building and maintaining an analytic practice. When the therapist greets the prospective patient at the door—and even before the first meeting, on the phone—her confidence and conviction, based on her respect for the analytic method, are what reach the patient.

The purpose of the first meeting and of the consultation phase in general is to decide whether patient and therapist can work together. This decision is based on different factors, some conscious and some unconscious. Each party assesses the other and part of the assessment is based on unconscious communication. Not much has been written on the match or the fit between patient and therapist although it determines the outcome of the work. Flarscheim (1972) talks about the therapist's ability to tolerate the patient's behavior in the office.

Since this depends on the ego state and psychopathology of the patient, *as well as the idiosyncratic personal interests and sensitivities of the particular therapist, it will not be the same for any two therapists.* A theo-

retical understanding widens our tolerance, as does a structured therapeutic setting, which defines the limits and responsibility of the therapist to the patient, thus expanding the freedom of the therapist to work
with whatever the patient brings to therapy. The therapist's own personal therapy can increase the range of conditions in which each individual therapist can function within an observational frame of reference. (p. 117, italics added)

These comments address important conscious material. Flarscheim's
focus on what the therapist can tolerate is crucial in the therapist's
decision to work with the patient. Beneath this ability is a less tan-
gible impression that I will call a "gut feeling" based on intuition. It
has to do with whether the therapist and the patient feel that they
can like each other, which is often based on unconscious transference feelings. The patient's manner, history, looks, and demeanor
imperceptibly register with the therapist, are usually intangible, and
always have an effect on the desire to work with this particular patient. If the therapist recognizes her reaction, thereby making it conscious, she has a choice about what to do to alter its impact. If the
disinclination to work with the patient is unconscious the therapist
will usually make an error or develop a blind spot that may ruin the
treatment possibilities right away or eventually. Every therapist has
unconscious feelings about every patient. Whether these feelings are
called countertransference or transference does not really matter as
much as how they are experienced and what is done with them. It is
hoped that the therapist will explore her initial reactions to the patient, whether positive or negative. It is important to remember that
the therapist's diagnostic impression can be influenced by her unconscious transference feelings, so that similarly trained therapists may
disagree on the patient's capacity to do analytic work. All of this is
inevitable and explains why the match is more important than the
diagnosis.

The next important step is gathering enough clinical data to form
diagnostic impressions, which the therapist then uses in order to form
a treatment plan to recommend to the patient. When reading an
article or book that sheds new light on a patient, it is sometimes dif-

ficult for the therapist to balance the intellectual knowledge gained with the ability to hear the patient's voice.

For instance, in determining a diagnosis the clinician is trained to look for different kinds of pathology, which includes ego defect, deficit, and deviation. Assessment of early ego development, structural defect, and recognition of character disorder, neurosis, borderline and narcissistic structures, schizoid behavior, schizophrenia, paranoia, and so on are required if one takes a psychiatric approach. Insurance companies require DSM diagnoses.

Another type of diagnosis is based on the developmental approach. Issues of separation-individuation and psychosexual development are assessed in order to determine fixation and regression. This requires an extensive history and an ability to make assumptions based on what the patient can tell us. Sometimes the patient's memory is clear, sometimes not. Usually it shifts over time, and basing a developmental diag- ❖ nosis on the information gained in the first meetings is imprecise. Many patients do not divulge certain information right away or even for several years. Childhood abuse and neglect is often not discussed or even remembered until the patient feels secure enough and trusts the therapist's ability to hear about traumatic issues in a calm, nonjudgmental way. Perverse behavior and fantasy is also often not talked about early in treatment.

Diagnostic or psychometric testing administered by a psychologist is not usually used by psychoanalytically oriented therapists because it is more useful for the therapist to learn about the patient through direct communication. Sending a patient for testing can split the transference, thereby threatening the integrity of the dyad.

The danger is that, with all of this important knowledge we can gather, we may cease to hear the even more important information, both conscious and unconscious, the patient has to convey both in words and in action over time.

A prospective patient, seen as a unique individual who has navigated her life in her own unique ways, will more likely feel respected than criticized or judged. She comes to the therapist when her own adaptations have become constricting, painful, or even unbearable and when she feels strong enough to seek help. I say "strong enough" because it does take strength to seek professional help. It is easier for many people to avoid, deny, and project their pain, to complain to friends or family, act out their feelings, and blame external forces. Bringing one's pain to a therapist means taking responsibility on some level, and this takes strength. Most people never cross the therapist's threshold. They have become inured to their ways of existing—and some seem to need the painful solutions that keep them going. The prospective patient, however, hopes for a second chance.

Although the knowledge the therapist gains through her education is crucial, it can sometimes deafen her to what the patient has to teach. Listening to patients with benign curiosity and without putting labels on them helps us learn to see what is between the lines of the literature and to learn to hear the unconscious communications along with the conscious ones. Labels are for clothes, not for people.

Borderline as a diagnostic category is confusing and not really helpful in deciding on a course of therapeutic action. Schizophrenic and manic-depressive or bi-polar disorder are categories that alert the therapist to discuss medication with a patient, but such labels say little in terms of the patient's ability to participate in psychoanalytically oriented treatment. Searles (1965) gives a moving example of a catatonic woman he treated at Chestnut Lodge. This patient did not speak for a very long time but Searles continued to see her for sessions regularly. When she did begin to speak she told him how important his patience was to her and that she remembered everything he had said. Giovacchini's book (1972) on treating the more disturbed patient is clear and convincing. Porder (1990) prescribes analytic work for the "sicker" patients. "Neurotics" are thought to be the patients most amenable to psychoanalytic treatment, however there are neurotic people who are extremely rigid and guarded, and unable to make use of therapy. Most neurotic people do not seek treatment, preferring to live with their obsessions and compulsions. And what often appears to be a neurotic structure is not. Even the labels sociopath or psychopath can cloud the picture in terms of treatment. What do these labels really mean? Is a person who lies or uses imposture to deal with anxiety not treatable or reachable?

Common sense in forming diagnostic impressions is not often mentioned in the literature but I believe it is really what matters most. When a patient mentions loss of a parent in childhood, an alcoholic parent, a family that moved a great deal, chronically ill parents, childhood illness, and other signs of trauma, the therapist listens for how these signs or events affected the patient. When an average expectable environment or good enough parenting is absent the security necessary for normal development is compromised. The therapist listens for how the patient adapted to and was affected by the past. As useful as training in psychoanalytic theory is, it must become the ground to the figure of the patient. This kind of posture or attitude requires patience, respect, and the ability not to know.

We can start now with the pressure we all have felt when a prospective patient makes the first appointment. One way to think about first meetings is to put oneself in the prospective patient's place. A therapist's first meeting with her own therapist is often the experience that is most influential in determining her behavior with a new patient. Feelings of anxiety, hopefulness, pain, and guardedness should be familiar to us, and this familiarity helps us empathize with the patient.

The initial phone contact makes an indelible impression on therapist and prospective patient. The tone of voice, manner of speaking, and what is said affect people in different ways. In some cases the first telephone contact greatly influences the patient's decision to continue with the therapist or to cancel the first appointment.

The first message the patient leaves and the first phone conversation often tell the two parties something about one another. If there is trouble reaching each other we register that. I have had messages where the person forgets to give her phone number. If the patient asks questions over the phone and cannot make an appointment unless answers are forthcoming the therapist senses the patient's anxiety. If the prospective patient can tolerate our wish not to respond over the phone, both parties learn something. The prospective patient hears the therapist set a boundary and the therapist sees that the caller is flexible enough to wait. A patient once told me towards the end of treatment that she felt safe from the first phone call. She felt that my not answering her questions made her feel that I knew what I was doing.

When I do reach the prospective patient I say, "Hello, this is Mrs. Hall returning your call." If she asks for an appointment I ask about her schedule (assuming I have more than one or two openings). If I can accommodate the patient's scheduling needs, I do. If not, I offer what I can. If a person can come only in the evening, for instance, and I have no evening hours available I say so and see if we can arrange something convenient to both of us. This interchange indicates something to the patient. Perhaps she notices that I tried to accommodate her. Perhaps she wonders if I am too busy to give her the attention she needs. Perhaps she feels reassured that I appear to be successful. If we cannot set up a mutually satisfactory time I ask if the person needs another name and, if so, I offer one. I also ask the caller if it is an emergency. If it is I try to accommodate her need for an immediate appointment by extending my day if possible. Sometimes the contact with the therapist on the phone can sustain a patient for a day or two. If the patient is desperate and I can't see her I offer another name immediately.

Things don't always go so smoothly. A patient may insist on answers over the phone. In such cases I say something like, "I understand that you are unsure about working with me but I think that meeting each other will serve your decision far more than my answering your questions on the phone." If it is a simple question and I can give a simple answer I will try but I haven't heard very many simple questions. One that comes to mind has to do with insurance and that one I try to answer. If a prospective patient inquires about my fee over the phone I tell her that we can talk about this in our first meeting. The explanation for this is that I have a range of fees and if a patient cannot afford my consultation fee I charge only what she can afford or nothing at all if that seems appropriate. I have found that if the two parties want to work together a suitable arrangement can usually be made. If not, the fee can be a way of escape. In such cases I do not offer a referral unless the patient requests one. The therapist usually has a list of colleagues or students who are building their practices and accept low fees. There are also excellent clinics in most areas.

Before we ever meet the prospective patient we have certain information. We are usually aware of the referral source and this in itself
can affect us. For instance, if a senior colleague or supervisor makes
the referral there is often the pressure of wanting to prove that we
are worthy. If the referral source gives a lot of information over the
phone we will find ourselves looking to verify or disprove what we
have been told. I try to discourage the referral source from giving me
a lot of information in a polite way. It is courteous, by the way, to let
the referral source know that the patient had an appointment and to
say thank you. This is all the information we can give because the
patient expects and deserves privacy. Sometimes a referring colleague
will ask how a patient they referred is working out. I don't feel comfortable answering the question because it infringes on the patient's
right to confidentiality. In order to be polite I usually thank the colleague again for thinking of me but express my discomfort in talking
about it. The same holds true when a colleague sees the relative of
my patient and wants to share information. I usually say something
like, "I think it would be less confusing and better in general not to
talk about it." Many therapists do discuss a case with the referral
source. I have found this confusing and unproductive. It is important
to see a patient as objectively as possible. Hearing someone else's
perceptions and opinions makes this difficult. Also, as psychoanalytically oriented clinicians we are bound to protect and preserve the
patient's right to confidentiality. Any breach of that promise puts us
at risk even more than the patient because when we break a promise
our work is compromised. Discussing a patient in supervision is the
only exception to this rule. In seminars or classes the therapist must
disguise the material when presenting a case.

If a patient wants me to see a family member or close friend I explore the patient's request as I do with any question. Exploring the
request usually helps the patient realize that referring to another
therapist would be best. I offer to make a referral if this is requested.
If the patient needs further explanation I merely say that another
therapist would be able to be completely neutral, impartial, unbi-
ased, and objective. I also might explain that it is important for me
to see the patient's friends and relatives through the patient's eyes

and meeting someone whom they talk about would make that difficult. Ultimately, the patient has the right to a therapist of her own.
This stance is difficult for someone who is trying to build a practice
but making referrals to colleagues is usually reciprocated. Close friends
are often thought of as siblings and therapists are often thought of as
parent figures. Treating a patient's close friend can exacerbate problems of sibling rivalry and often increases the patient's temptation to
act out by talking outside of treatment about things that have their
place in treatment. In a very small community this policy may be
impractical. In such cases the therapist might explain to the patients
that talking about one's treatment with someone else can lead to
complications and is best avoided. (At any time during treatment
when we hear that a patient is talking to others about her treatment
or sharing dreams with others before telling the therapist we should
explore why and tell the patient that this can complicate treatment.)
These issues are related to first meetings because they often come up
during the consultation phase and it's comforting to both parties to
be clear about policy from the start.

When the therapist sees a couple for marital counseling and then
realizes that individual treatment is the treatment of choice she must
decide which patient to refer out or whether to refer both parties to
different therapists. If the therapist finds that she would prefer to work
with one or the other of the couple she would do well to examine
her intuition and follow it if she is clear about her decision. The therapist can also ask the couple to decide. The person she decides to refer
will feel rejection or possibly relief but these feelings can and should
be explored by the next therapist. This holds true for all referrals.
The therapist who receives a referral from another therapist who has
seen the patient, even once, must be alert to and listen for feelings of
rejection. The patient's anger at the first therapist will usually be trans-
ferred to the new therapist.

It is important to be clear about one's policy regarding charging
for the initial consultation. A supervisee told me about a patient who
had been given eight referrals. The prospective patient was surprised
that she would be charged for the consultation because none of the
other people she had consulted charged her. The therapist's policy

was to charge for consultations and he was sure he would not be chosen. He was surprised when the patient began treatment with him. My reading of this situation is that the therapist stated his professional requirements in a nonthreatening, respectful manner and that this impressed the patient. Patients sense insecurity quickly and because this therapist knew himself, and was able to convey his policy and not change it to compete with others, the patient felt safe.

This applies to policies regarding fee, billing, and payment practice and charging for missed sessions. Once therapist and patient decide to work together the therapist's requirements must be stated (see Chapter 1). I say to the patient that my fee is X. I then ask if this is feasible for her. If not and if I can lower the fee I explain that I have a sliding scale and that we can begin at Y with the understanding that the fee will change as her income increases. I then tell the patient that I give a bill at the end of the month and expect to be paid in the first week of the following month. I tell the patient that she is responsible for her hours even if she is unable to come to therapy. I also tell the patient that I take certain time off (usually three or four weeks in August and two weeks in the spring or winter) and that I may attend a conference each year. I tell the patient that I give several months' notice and that I hope we can coordinate our vacations so that therapy can proceed with as few interruptions as possible. These conditions sound unfair to some patients and if the patient complains I explain my rationale. I also use the reactions to help us understand the objections.

Different therapists have different policies. If we remember that consistency and reliability are crucial in allowing the patient to trust, we will find it possible to be firm about our policies, whatever they are. Flexibility, though important, can seem like insecurity to a beginning patient. Limits and boundaries provide a safe structure. A student told me that a patient was upset about her policy for charging for missed sessions so the student agreed to excuse the patient for five sessions each year. The patient never came back. Backing down because of a patient's anger about a policy rather than exploring it gives the patient the message that we are not comfortable with anger. Such a message insures the failing of a major test (see Chapter 7).

The way we greet questions is important, and I have found that a welcoming, professional stance is more important than any answers we may give. As I said in Chapter 1, it is usually not helpful to answer personal questions but a reason for this stance is in order. I say something like, "Your questions are valuable and important because they will help us understand you. It would be easy for me to answer but more helpful to you if you say what comes to mind."

Questions about the therapist's credentials or training or type of therapy practiced should be answered in the consultation period, especially if they are asked genuinely. If they are asked sarcastically or belligerently this should be addressed. A patient once said, "You're not Freudian, are you?" I said that I would answer the question but asked her to tell me what she meant first. She said that her understanding was that if I were a Freudian I would never speak and if I did it would be about her sex life. I replied that I was a psychoanalyst, that Freud was the father of psychoanalysis, that there would be a lot to talk about besides sex, and that I might not talk a lot, especially before I got to know her, but when I felt I could contribute I certainly would. I would also note the patient's sarcasm because such a question could be asked benignly. I might say, "You asked in what seemed an angry tone. Can you tell me about that?"

The therapist's courtesy and calmness get her through some difficult situations. Several minutes before the time is up I tell the prospective patient that we will be stopping shortly. If I feel another consultation is necessary to clarify or learn more before we decide to work together, I suggest another appointment. The therapist may know within the first few minutes of a consultation that intensive treatment is what's needed but this perception may frighten some patients away. I say something like, "Let's arrange another appointment to talk more and decide what the best course of action is." If the patient is depressed, has suffered a recent loss, or is in a state of high anxiety I offer another appointment within a day or two. If the therapist knows that she cannot work with the patient for whatever reason she should make that clear as quickly as possible and offer a referral if appropriate. If the patient presents unusual or dangerous symptoms in the first consultation appointment the therapist will usually want to schedule the next appointment within the week, or even on the next day if possible.

> Miss Long had been experiencing intense anxiety for some weeks before her first appointment. During the session she was able to articulate her fears and seemed to calm down a bit. The therapist felt that a connection was made and suggested they meet on the following day. The patient expressed relief and treatment continued on a daily (weekday) basis. When there was some understanding of the anxiety and when it abated patient and therapist discussed a treatment plan.

What if the patient is not able to afford the therapist's fee? Common sense tells us that a referral must be made as quickly as possible.

Because each patient is unique, each first meeting is different. However, there are some similarities in the way I try to conduct a first session and I will begin by discussing these.

When I open the door to greet the prospective patient I say something like, "Mr. X? I'm Mrs. Hall," and offer my hand. I like to shake hands on first meeting because I have experienced the handshake as a welcoming gesture that breaks the ice. It sets a formal, professional, warm tone. If the therapist shares a waiting room and there are others sitting in it she must announce who she is first so as to honor the prospective patient's privacy.

I invite the person into my office and motion to the chair. All of these details sound quite elementary but I have been surprised at how many beginning therapists welcome this information. I believe that everyone must develop her own style and I am sharing my style here.

Many psychoanalysts treat the initial interview as they would treat an analytic session. This makes sense when the patient has come for analysis. When the patient does not know about psychoanalysis such an approach may feel offensive or even traumatic. The therapist uses her clinical judgment and common sense based on the patient. Perhaps to compensate for the more old-fashioned analytic stance of silence in the beginning of a first interview some analysts go the other way.

> Mr. Marshall consulted an analyst who was welcoming and warm but who overstepped his professional boundaries. The prospective patient was a musician and the analyst told him what musicians he admired. Mr. Marshall realized that the analyst was being friendly but found his comments out of place. He did not return.

There are different ways to start the first meeting. Some analysts are silent and wait for the patient to begin. If you can do that it is helpful in informing the patient that this is her space and that she has the freedom to use it as she chooses. The opening remarks can tell both parties a lot. Whatever the patient begins with must of course be greeted by attentive listening. If the analyst feels she can use the patient's beginning approach to deepen the work by making an observation that shows the patient something new or makes her feel understood this is desirable.

> Mr. Field began by talking of how difficult it was to get to the session due to traffic. He went on to express his relief that he made the appointment on time. He said he was always prompt and usually early for appointments. After more along the same lines the therapist wondered aloud if it was also difficult to seek therapy.

This "wondering" accomplished several things: (1) the patient heard a tone of interest and understanding; (2) the patient was indeed having trouble getting started and this comment made it easier to begin; (3) the patient heard the therapist "wonder" and it introduced the idea of not knowing but finding out.

I usually say something to put a new person at relative ease. "So." "What brings you?" "Can you tell me about yourself?" are benign starters that, combined with an attentive posture and facial expression, usually make it easy for the person to begin. Some therapists sit with a pad ready to make notes. I prefer to listen. I have found that taking notes sparingly when a person is giving a history that includes sibling order and other details is necessary for me. But in the first hour I am more interested in my impressions of the prospective patient and in establishing rapport. There is always time to go back to details once a rapport is in place. I also like to leave time for the prospective patient's questions. I try to schedule consultations at the end of the day or before a break so as not to feel rushed. I do, however, stick as close to the 45 minutes as possible.

John Klauber (1972) advocates a longer first interview and asks for specific information. Phyllis Greenacre (1956) believed in taking an extensive history in the first interviews. I have found that 45 or 50 minutes is comfortable for both parties and I prefer a more open-ended approach. A patient will usually tell the therapist why she has come. Common reasons for seeking therapy are recent loss, marital difficulties, inability to sustain relationships and/or jobs, illness in one's family, and other stressful and depressing situations. Sometimes a person complains of vague disappointment in life, lack of energy, or feeling stuck or blocked. All of these reasons have roots. How does the therapist begin to assess the patient's need for and ability to use psychoanalytic work? What questions can we ask that help us learn about the strength or fragility, the autonomous functioning or the inability to function independently, and the psychological-mindedness of the patient?

Asking the patient to tell us something about her childhood or life at home when she was growing up can tell us something about the patient's resilience, ego strength, possible abuse or neglect, and ability to self-regulate. I usually say something like, "Can you tell me something about where you grew up?" or "How many in your family?" or "Where did you go to school?" One of these questions usually gets the ball rolling.

If the patient gets involved in talking about her reason for coming, I listen and wait for an appropriate time to ask about history. I always ask if the patient has been in therapy before. If the answer is yes, I ask about it. Information about prior treatment gives the therapist an idea of what worked, what did not work, and what the chances are of becoming one of a string of failed therapists. I try to get a sense of why previous treatment did not last and I frequently ask how the patient imagines this treatment will help.

At some point in the consultation phase I inquire about early child-hood illness or loss. Sheldon Bach (personal communication) often asks the patient to tell about what it was like at bedtime. If the patient had no bedtime and no assistance or routine at bedtime the therapist can determine that she was not regulated by a parental fig-ure. This knowledge clues us in to areas of trauma and neglect and alerts us to possible consequences.

Gertrude Blanck (personal communication) sometimes asked the patient about memories of birthdays. Such memories can give the therapist an idea about how parental figures treated special occasions in the patient's childhood.

> Miss Trent grew up in an affluent family but was largely ignored in terms of bedtime, homework, and mealtimes. Her parents seemed to love her but they were too preoccupied to pay enough attention. When visiting a friend she was expected to finish her milk, something that never hap-pened at home. Birthdays were celebrated at camp, never at home. She became a performer, for she thought that this was her best chance of getting attention. Since the audience could never make up for her early childhood deprivation, she continued to feel empty and lonely.

Pictures such as these can tell the therapist a great deal about a patient but she must be cautious. It is important to remember that a patient's view of her history usually changes, sometimes drastically, during the course of treatment. Many patients begin by painting rosy pictures of the past. "My mother was a saint, my father an angel, childhood was fun," are variations on a theme. Often parents are depicted one-sidedly in the opposite direction. Gradually, as the patient starts to look inside, and as she feels safe with the nonjudg-mental therapist, things begin to shift.

A particularly moving example of a shift in the opposite direction can be found in Jill Herbert's paper, "The Haunted Analysis" (1997). Her patient, Mr. A., spoke early in treatment of the family atmosphere as "sterile and blank, maintaining that this meagerness accounted, in large part, for his problems and sufferings" (p. 194). He spoke of his father as "unimportant . . . an embarrassment, awkward and socially inept" (p. 194). Mr. A.'s mother was described as ". . . nothing. She never worked and she stayed home. The house was empty. The TV was always on. We never did anything as a family, never went anywhere" (p. 194). Years later patient and analyst witnessed the power of fantasy in distorting memory. It emerged that Mr. A.'s father was a successful business executive who with his wife took an active part in community life. "The family took vacations together skiing, boating, and travelling while weekends were taken up with country club social activities. The house was often filled with many friends of the adults and of the four children" (p. 203).

Examples like this teach the analytically oriented therapist to keep an open mind and to avoid carving her patients' memories and perceptions in stone. Early pictures of the past are bound to shift over time. Diagnostic impressions based on the first history will change as the history changes. For example, a patient with intense oedipal jealousy and rage casts her mother in an evil light. The mother's ability to tolerate her daughter's normal wishes for her disappearance does much to determine the outcome of their relationship. Ms. Briggs in Chapter 8 is an example of how memories of a mother can change during analysis.

Early pictures of a patient, if taken by the therapist with appropriate grains of sugar and salt, will change as treatment takes hold. The analytically minded therapist learns to wait patiently. Therapists trained in more active forms of therapy are more inclined to work with the first pictures presented and to take sides against the "villains" and for the "heroes." For instance, Miss Anthony complained continuously about her sister, whom she described as intrusive and selfish. Examples were given that sounded convincing. The behavior therapist actively takes her patient's side by suggesting specific tactics that could be used to confront and control the sister. The analytic therapist tries to interest the patient in expressing her own feelings by saying something like, "It seems really hard for you to deal with this situation. Can you tell more about how you feel?" "Has it always been this way?"

Clinicians are taught that diagnosis should inform the therapist as to what treatment mode is appropriate. Historically, it has been taught that psychoanalysis is the treatment of choice for the "neurotic," and that psychotherapy is the treatment of choice for the "borderline" and "psychotic." The reasons for this include such statements as: the borderline patient does not differentiate between self and object; the patient whose ego is not intact has trouble tolerating the frustrations imposed by the abstinent analyst; there is not sufficient repression in the borderline; failure in the separation-individuation phase makes it impossible for the patient to recognize the analyst as a separate object, thereby precluding the development of a transference neurosis; borderline rage threatens to destroy the object and should not be permitted.

Such sweeping statements, correct as they may be at certain times, can tend to make our perception of a patient more rigid than is useful, just as certain descriptions of psychoanalysis or "classical analysis" are rigid and unrealistic and serve to frighten us, the patient, and the public away. Our perceptions and assessments of our patients must be made over time and with their individuality foremost in our minds. As I mentioned earlier, each patient must write his or her own theory and each therapist must be willing to let the treatment deepen. Anna Freud (Freud et al. 1965) said that we cannot know the diagnosis until the end of treatment.

I do not mean that knowledge of metapsychology, oedipal and pre-oedipal conflict, masochism and sadism, fixation and regression, annihilation, separation and castration anxiety, and individuation issues, along with Kleinian, Freudian, object relations, and self psychology theories of technique are not important. But we must feel free to listen for how such theoretical constructs and techniques fit and are experienced by each patient we treat.

Porder (1990), in an excellent paper in the book On Beginning an Analysis on "Beginning with Borderline Patients," requires the "sicker" patient to agree to a four-to-five-times-a-week analysis. Porder does not believe in categorizing patients according to a borderline diagnosis because there is such a wide range of pathology in a group which "lies somewhere between psychosis, on the more seriously disturbed end of the spectrum, and neurosis or neurotic character on the healthier end" (p. 163). His paper addresses itself to the treatment of sicker patients who come to the office practice of psycho-analytically trained psychotherapists or psychoanalysts. These patients live severely chaotic lives, with self-destructive tendencies and poor reality testing. After taking a history and assessing the patient's ego functioning Porder proposes an essentially analytic treatment. "I explain to the patient the rule of free association and the relative inactivity and neutrality of the analyst. . . . I recommend that we meet for sessions four to five times a week, and explain that I recommend this frequency because of the chronicity and the fixity of their emotional problems. I realize that this means there is a significant self-selection among my patients, since those who are too frightened will not continue with me" (p. 164).

While I agree with Porder's prescription for treatment I believe in telling the patient who refuses this contract something like, "From what you have told me I think you would find four or five times a week most helpful but we can begin where you feel most comfortable. Hopefully, you will increase your sessions as you begin to understand the work." This is a controversial approach and it has its pitfalls. The patient may sense that you are fearful of working with her, or that you have reservations about her prognosis, as indeed you may have. My hope is that the patient will respond to my willingness to work with her, my confidence in the process, and also my consideration of her pace (see Chapters 4 and 5).

Another problem arises in prescribing for the "sicker" patient. The therapist often does not find out until after the patient begins to trust her (and this can take years) about self-destructive or perverse behavior.

Mrs. Skye, (see also Chapter 7) told the therapist about her self-cutting after several years of twice-a-week therapy. The therapist's ability to remain calm and benignly curious permitted Mrs. Skye to explore what this meant by looking at when it occurred and figuring out how she was feeling at the time. When Mrs. Skye began with her therapist she found it impossible to commit to twice-a-week treatment. Her gradual and growing trust permitted her to share alarming problems over time and to increase the frequency of her sessions.

Mrs. Skye would be considered a "sicker" patient by Porder and by others but she would not have agreed to more than once-a-week sessions at the start of therapy. It was necessary for her to make sure the therapist was trustworthy. In this case the therapist brought up the issue of increasing sessions whenever she heard a reference, even obliquely, to the patient's need for more time.

Many therapists I meet in supervision or in the classroom gain their experience in clinics, as I did. If the clinic administrator or supervisor is aware that the therapist is in training she often gives permission for treatment to be conducted twice or three times a week (see Chapter 5). In such cases the therapist can tell the patient in the first interview that work is best done two or more times a week.

Another issue to think about regarding the more disturbed patient is our role as therapist. Sometimes our fantasies of rescue loom larger than is appropriate, and sometimes we become unduly frightened. Patients test our comfort in our role as neutral, nonjudgmental, concerned professionals who believe in promoting autonomy and in understanding the roots of troubling lives. Adult patients deserve to be treated as such. It can be argued that their reality testing and capacity to exercise good judgment is faulty, even dangerous, but, as Ella Sharpe (1950) said, we are not reformers or educators. We are skilled in psychoanalytic treatment and if we keep within those boundaries we will do our best work. All this is to say that on first meeting a prospective patient we will do best if we think of the work ahead as collaborative. If the prospective patient can join us our chances of success are greater. Sometimes it takes years for a collaboration to evolve and in such cases the therapist must be willing and able to be patient. Coming to sessions must be seen as an effort to collaborate even if the patient seems uninvolved otherwise.

Other approaches to assessing a patient's readiness for psychoanalytic work are Winnicott's (1954) therapeutic diagnoses: Can the patient sustain herself outside of treatment and get to her appointments, and can she behave in a way during sessions that the therapist finds tolerable? Klauber (1972) takes a cautious and conservative approach towards recommending analytic work. He sees analysis as an enormous investment of hope and lists types of patients he is wary of. These include mothers with an infant in the suburbs, people with psychosomatic symptoms, and charming patients.

It is agreed that psychoanalysis is an investment of hope, but the philosophy on which this book is based is that people have a right to be naturally curious about themselves, especially when their functioning is compromised by conflict and derailed development. Psychoanalytic work provides a person with space and time to grow and to resolve conflict. If patients are motivated to change and to grow, whether charming or plagued with psychosomatic symptoms, they have a right to take the psychoanalytic journey. A patient who has an infant in the suburbs may have the ability to make suitable arrangements that permit her to come to analysis. It is not the therapist's decision but the patient's autonomous right to decide. Klauber also advocates sharing information with family members who financially support treatment. It is a breach of confidentiality to share clinical material (unless suicidal or homicidal plans are being made.) When the patient's family pays for treatment, I bill the patient and ask her to pay me directly. I explain that our work is strictly between us and that even receiving payment from an outside source can threaten the work. For the same reason I do not accept direct payment from insurance companies and ask the patient to arrange to be reimbursed by the company and to pay me directly. Sometimes a parent will set up a special account for the patient or arrange to pay the patient so that she can be responsible for paying her bills. This policy guards against contaminating the transference and promotes the patient's autonomy.

Rothstein (1994) does not try to measure a patient in terms of analyzability. He approaches each consultation with an optimistic attitude as to the patient's aptitude for analysis and he emphasizes that "if any particularly positive, hopeful, negative, or pessimistic ideas about the patient, the diagnosis, or the prognosis occur to me during a consultation, I view it as possibly reflective of an emerging counter-transference–transference engagement" (p. 683). He goes on to say, "Conjectures about diagnosis that carry a negative valence, such as borderline, narcissistic, psychopathic, or perverse, may signal such a countertransference trend" (p. 684).

Diagnostic approaches require the therapist to be on the lookout for something. If these diagnostic approaches are combined with the stance of benevolent curiosity and neutral observation the therapist's ability to prescribe an appropriate treatment plan and to let the treatment deepen is enhanced. The goal is to synthesize one's training in theory and technique (not that we ever stop learning), making it into the ground and letting the patient stand out as the figure. The information that informs diagnosis is important in shaping the therapist's approach to a patient but if the diagnosis overshadows the treatment possibilities it can blind and deafen us to the intricacies and subtleties of our patients. People are too complex to be categorized. The idea of *diagnostic impressions* is more useful and saves us from labeling a patient. Impressions are easier to alter than labels.

After the first session or sessions, based on my diagnostic impressions and my gut feeling about the patient, and if I feel hopeful that we can work together, I lay out the options. I mention during the first consultation that psychoanalytic work is done from two to five times a week and that the couch makes sense for many people because it has a freeing effect. I have found that mentioning the possibilities early in treatment is nonthreatening and respectful of the patient's autonomy. If a patient insists on once-a-week treatment I will usually begin that way with the understanding that we reevaluate the frequency issue as we progress. I also do my best to explain the value of more frequent sessions. If the patient is clearly in need of and able to benefit from analysis without preliminary work I tell her that this is the treatment of choice during the consultation phase of treatment. For instance, a woman in her thirties who consulted me had been in therapy before, once and twice a week for two years. Her analyst had given her much intellectual insight but she was perplexed and in pain. My assessment was that due to her psychological-mindedness, her problems, and her prior experience, analysis was the treatment of choice. She accepted the recommendation and we began analysis immediately. Other patients need to go more slowly.

As mentioned earlier, it is important to know the patient's treatment history. If a patient has been to many therapists the chances are good that the list of failed treatments will grow. The patient's reasons for ending previous treatments should be explored thoroughly during the consultation phase and understood before a new treatment is begun.

If the patient is seriously ill, obviously self-destructive, experiencing panic or high anxiety, I tell her plainly and simply that once a week will be of little or of no use and that two or more times a week is a minimum requirement. I try to straddle the line between firmness and flexibility because some patients are too frightened to commit to more than once a week and need the opportunity to test the waters by wading in. I think that a patient is more likely to consider the therapist's recommendation when it is made with respect and explanation. Telling a patient that she must be seen a specific number of times a week invites a power struggle or compliance. Telling the patient what is optimal and necessary is not as off-putting. The therapist's confidence and willingness to treat are always being tested. Most patients quickly register timidity and tiptoeing on the therapist's part. If the therapist states what she feels is required with conviction the patient will feel comfortable—even though the patient may not agree and may need to test the waters first.

Porder (1990) proposes an "essentially analytic contract" to the sicker patient. He explains his recommendation for four- or five-times-a-week treatment by addressing the patient at her highest level. Porder does not treat those people who do not agree to his prescription for treatment.

This book presents clinical material to support a "testing the waters" approach when a patient is not ready or able to commit to four or five times a week.

Some things we learn about a person in the first meeting are:

1. Levels of anxiety. (Does the anxiety diminish or increase during the session?);
2. Access to affect;
3. Level of appropriateness;
4. Potential for humor;
5. Ability to look inside or to question one's motives (psychological-mindedness);

6. Need to externalize;
7. Level of patience;
8. Ability to be flexible;
9. Defenses favored. (If a patient's history sounds traumatic in any way I listen for how the patient reacted in the past and how she views her reaction today);
10. Ability to include the therapist. (Anxious patients and patients with histories of intrusive parents often flood the therapist, making it impossible for her to get a word in.)

Sometimes the therapist is thrown off balance in a first meeting. The patient who exhibits unusual or inappropriate behavior, the extremely silent patient, the patient who brings her lunch and proceeds to eat it during the session are a few situations that occur to me.

One of my first clinic patients told me in the initial interview that he had a garbage machine in his head and, opening his mouth, asked me if I could hear it. I was a student and not at all prepared for this situation so I listened, said no, and asked him to tell me about himself. Where did he grow up, who did he live with, and so on. He answered my questions and a beginning rapport was established. Focusing him seemed to allay some of his anxiety. We later came to understand that the garbage machine stood for unacceptable thoughts. His initial behavior was his way of saying, "I'm a frightened person with dirty thoughts. Will you be afraid of and disgusted by me?" My benign curiosity and common sense carried me through an unusual situation.

The main goal of the first meeting or meetings is to have more meetings. These are far more likely to occur when respect and benevolent curiosity overshadow the need for labels.

❖ C H A P T E R   3 ❖

Deepening
the Treatment

Once the therapist has set the stage for psychoanalytic work and has passed the initial tests, once the two parties have sized each other up and a beginning rapport has been established, deepening the treatment becomes the therapist's focus. By deepening the treatment I mean engaging the patient in looking beneath the surface, thereby expanding her understanding of what makes her tick. I will illustrate the process by introducing Mr. Lopez.

Mr. Lopez came to a clinic for therapy at age 21 as a condition of probation. He had been arrested for selling drugs on campus at the college he was attending. He initially viewed therapy as a way of avoiding jail. His probation term was five years. The therapist was not expected to report to the probation officer but if asked was expected to verify attendance. (This never happened.)

In adolescence Mr. Lopez began smoking marijuana and went on to experiment with both soft and hard drugs at college. While using drugs was a definite part of the culture at the time, selling drugs became more satisfying for him. It provided him with the self-esteem and identity he sought. Being important and powerful was the high he became addicted to.

Mr. Lopez's parents came to this country from Cuba, and the long, hard hours they worked in their restaurant left little time or energy for raising their six children. Mr. Lopez, the youngest by ten years, was alternately spoiled and neglected as a child. Because his parents were rarely home to supervise and set limits, Mr. Lopez felt abandoned, lonely, and deprived, but when his mother was home he felt coddled, entitled, and smothered. He described himself in childhood as a tyrant with no discipline. Mr. Lopez was highly intelligent and did well academically. His teachers either hated or loved him. His strong need for attention was either gratified or rebuffed by them.

He remembered his behavior in school as either endearing or disruptive. He was calling for attention while at the same time pushing it away.

Mr. Lopez began once-a-week therapy, saying that he would fulfill his probation requirement but didn't see the point of therapy. His therapist said she understood that he saw therapy as a must but thought he might find it an interesting process. Later in treatment Mr. Lopez reflected on the first sessions and said he found the therapist's hopefulness relieving. He also remembered the therapist's calm way of talking and was impressed by her interest in what he had to say. No one had ever listened to him without arguing or judging him before. After several sessions Mr. Lopez said he would use therapy to "get it all together, to have different interests and to get to know Gilberto Lopez." In the first month of treatment Mr. Lopez shifted his attitude towards therapy and articulated his wish for a "second chance."

What happened to effect the change in Mr. Lopez's attitude? His therapist conveyed her interest, respect, patience, and hopefulness by her nonjudgmental and attentive demeanor, and by her benevolent curiosity (see Chapter 1). It was not just what she said to Mr. Lopez, it was how she genuinely felt. Her thoughts ran like this: *Here is a young man who had a difficult and lonely childhood (empathy). He's in trouble (benevolent curiosity). He is here in my office (hopefulness); He has a story to tell (interest); He survived (respect). I like him.*

Empathy, interest, hopefulness, and the ability to like the patient set a tone of acceptance that is felt and responded to by the patient. It is the therapist's attitude more than her words that conveys the message. In fact, if the attitude of respect and hopefulness is missing, words will mean nothing. This is what I mean by unconscious communication and gut feeling. The therapist's attitude determines her ability to use psychoanalytic technique effectively. Hearing and interpreting resistance, transference, acting out, enactment, dreams, associations, and silence (making sense out of the patient's communication and lack of communication) rest on the therapist's knowledge of unconscious processes, an ability to be hopeful, and a basic ability to like the patient.

Mr. Lopez began his fourth session by reporting the memory of a fight at age 12 with a neighborhood kid who said Mr. Lopez's parents didn't love him because they were never home. Mr. Lopez remembered fighting because he felt hurt. In looking back he felt it was true. In college he felt comfortable by being cool and unemotional. Here, he was giving the therapist a glimpse of the work ahead. He was telling the therapist that he could be very demanding and could cover his neediness by seeming not to care. He was also testing to see if she would be judgmental by agreeing that his behavior was bad. After a while, Mr. Lopez became silent. The therapist took this opportunity to tell him that he would learn about himself by saying whatever came to mind, even if he had thoughts that seemed not to relate to the subject he had been talking about. Mr. Lopez responded by saying, "The world is round." The therapist waited quietly and eventually Mr. Lopez began commenting on things in the office. He expressed some discomfort by challenging the relevancy of what he had said. The therapist said, "If you follow your thoughts they will lead you somewhere, and you will learn about yourself." Mr. Lopez shrugged and said that the mind was really complex. He smiled as the session ended.

Introducing the patient to the idea of free association is really quite simple and natural. If it is done in a gentle and thoughtful way and if it makes sense to the patient he feels accepted and encouraged. Mr. Lopez felt a lifting of the pressure to perform. He also heard that his therapist was interested in whatever he had to say, whether it made sense or not. This does not mean that the patient will associate freely at all times. In future sessions Mr. Lopez spoke of feeling blocked or of his mind going blank. This often means that thoughts about the therapist are going on. The therapist can say, at such times, something like, "Usually when your mind goes blank or you feel blocked about saying something it means you are having thoughts about me." I have found that such an explanation gives the patient permission to talk more freely about the therapist. Many patients will say, "I didn't think my thoughts about you were part of therapy." Other patients say, "As a matter of fact, I was wondering . . ." I have never heard a patient complain about this information/permission, which serves to deepen the treatment. Patients frequently have conscious thoughts about the therapist, especially in the beginning of treatment. Later in treatment the analyst listens to the patient's material with an ear for the indirect expression of transference. For instance, if the therapist has announced a separation or vacation and the patient begins talking about how angry or upset he is with his boss the therapist can ask if the patient is having angry feelings towards her. I might say something like, "I wonder if your anger at the boss also applies to me." If the patient denies recognition of anger or upset at the therapist, she can explain that in announcing a break in treatment she is like a boss who makes the rules or calls the shots without consulting the employee.

In the following session Mr. Lopez spoke about his father's illness and death and connected his fear of "not getting it all" before it was too late. He worried about dying young. He remembered crying when he first learned about death when he was 4. At the end of the session he asked if he could come to therapy twice instead of once a week. After exploring his request the therapist said she would let him know when there was an opening in her schedule.

In following sessions the theme was instant gratification. The patient said that part of him wanted instant happiness and a perfect life and that part of him knew there was no such thing and that the latter part questioned the former part. The therapist connected his wishes to the previous session and the therapist's not granting his request for more sessions per week immediately.

The capacity to have mixed feelings was an indication of conflict and Mr. Lopez's ability to question his thoughts indicated an observing ego. The therapist used this information to form diagnostic impressions. Other impressions were based on Mr. Lopez's difficult childhood, inconsistent parenting, his difficulty tolerating frustration, his faulty judgment (which led to selling drugs), and his mistrust of teachers. The therapist was impressed by Mr. Lopez's intelligence, sense of humor, resilience, and psychological-mindedness. One could say that therapist and patient were assessing and testing each other.

As treatment progressed and Mr. Lopez felt engaged and "into it" he began to regress. He wanted the therapist to meet his mother, to give him more time, and to call him by his first name. He was angry at not getting his way but at the same time he made it clear that he valued his treatment and the therapist's ability to provide boundaries. These boundaries were tested vigorously over time because Mr. Lopez had rarely been given limits. He acted out his anger at the therapist for setting limits and for not arranging to see him twice a week immediately by fighting with his roommate. The therapist told him that his actions reflected his anger at her. After this interpretation Mr. Lopez asked if he could swear in therapy.

Regression is to be expected in psychoanalytic work. Along with transference it is the key to understanding the past and how it affects the present. The past is repeated in the present with the therapist as ● transference object and as a new object. Loewald (1960) in his paper "On The Therapeutic Action of Psychoanalysis" explains the process:

> Analysis is thus understood as an intervention designed to set ego development in motion, be it from a point of relative arrest, or to promote what we conceive of as a healthier direction. . . . This is achieved by the promotion and utilization of (controlled) regression. . . . The transference neurosis, in the sense of re-activation of the childhood neurosis, is set in motion not simply by the technical skill of the analyst, but by the fact that the analyst makes himself available for the development of a new "object-relationship" between the patient and the analyst. The patient tends to make this potentially new object-relationship into an old one. . . . The patient can dare to take the plunge into the regressive crisis of the transference neurosis which brings him face to face again with his childhood anxieties and conflicts, if he can hold on to the potentiality of a new object-relationship, represented by the analyst. [p. 224]

The term *transference neurosis* is usually reserved for psychoanalysis proper but in many cases of psychoanalytic psychotherapy taking place twice or even once a week the patient does become involved with the therapist on an intense level that is based not on present reality but on past scenarios. I have heard analysts call this a *psychotic transference* and I disagree. Usually these patients have less rigid defenses and regress more quickly than those with a more neurotic (well-defended) structure. These patients are seen as having a borderline structure that indicates trouble differentiating self and object. Differentiating self and object is not an all or nothing-at-all process, however. In times of stress and anxiety such differentiation can ebb defensively. These difficulties do not add up to a psychotic transference—a term, like other labels, that cuts off exploration. An analogy that occurs to me is that of a car with good shock absorbers as opposed to one with less effective shock absorbers. With the latter the ride is bumpier. Both cars work and can travel the necessary distance but one journey will be smoother than the other. When traveling on a smooth road the difference is not necessarily felt at all. One common result of treatment is more effective shock absorbers.

In the first few sessions a patient will often present his highest level of functioning. This is helpful, for it shows the therapist what has been achieved in terms of ego development and ability to relate to another person. (Sometimes a patient will present florid symptomology or disorganization in a first interview due to high anxiety. As the anxiety abates a higher level of functioning and organization often becomes apparent.) The nature of the analytic atmosphere and the regular meetings between patient and therapist are conducive to (controlled) regression and to the manifestations of transference.

A child's ability to pretend and play act is an important way of communication that reemerges in treatment. As treatment progresses, the patient begins to see that the therapist has no fast answers or solutions, and that the work involves looking inside and to the past in order to make sense of the present. By monitoring the ways the patient thinks and feels about the therapist and by paying attention to the patient's relations with the outside world, which reflect past attitudes being acted out in the present (the transference and the tendency to repeat), the therapeutic dyad begins to see patterns. Making sense of the patterns is one goal of psychoanalytic work.

Mr. Lopez began to express hatred of his mother and, for the first time, empathy for his father. He felt that his mother acted like a child and he had to be the adult. With feeling he reported how his mother had leaned on him both emotionally and physically during his father's illness and after his death when Mr. Lopez was 17. His older siblings had left home and had families of their own. He spent a session remembering his father, whom he saw as a depressed man. Father's illness began when the patient was 12. There were operations and periods of convalescence during which Mr. Lopez felt guilty and frightened.

The therapist began to have an idea of how the transference would develop. Mr. Lopez would bring his anger, frustration, yearnings, and mistrust into the treatment with the therapist as recipient of these and other feelings. With a history of neglect and overindulgence the treatment is usually a stormy one because the rage is intense.

During the first four months of once-a-week therapy Mr. Lopez's history unfolded naturally and with much appropriate affect. Learning about a patient's childhood history is meaningful to both therapist and patient, especially when it unfolds naturally. Taking a detailed history during the consultation phase is exactly that: a taking. Both therapist and patient learn far more when it emerges in the patient's own time and at his own pace. A person's history is never completely or accurately given because memories are recovered in their own time and because as the treatment progresses things are seen differently—in three dimensions and living color. A history given in the first few sessions can be helpful to the therapist (Chapter 2) but it is usually one-dimensional because it is given at the therapist's request and before any trust has developed. Analytic work is best done without direction. A patient cannot be expected to tell embarrassing and shameful things to someone unless he can be relatively sure that he will not be judged. This takes time for many people and it means testing and retesting the safety of the waters.

One day, after a particularly difficult session filled with memories of his father's death, for which he felt responsible in some way, Mr. Lopez came close to throwing a book. He left the session abruptly and came back in a few minutes to apologize. He saw that the therapist was not about to retaliate and instead invited him to finish his session. Mr. Lopez later told the therapist that this incident was a milestone for him for two reasons: not throwing the book meant that he had more control than he realized, and he saw that the therapist remained calm. A test from both sides had been passed and Mr. Lopez felt safe enough to deepen the treatment by sharing more material. The therapist learned that Mr. Lopez was volatile but not violent, and the patient learned that the therapist could remain calm and nonjudgmental.

In the fifth month of therapy Mr. Lopez began coming twice a week. More frequent contact helped him bring more anger and frustration into treatment. Instead of fighting with friends and relatives he began attacking his therapist verbally. "Why can't you know what I'm thinking?" "Why can't I have primal scream therapy?" "You don't know anything." "Why can't you help me?" This tantrum ran its course and Mr. Lopez associated to how dependent his mother was after his father's death. He had to be the adult, pick out her shoes, hold her up at his father's funeral. And now she was seeing another man who was taking her time. Mr. Lopez was jealous and furious at losing his place of importance. He admitted having felt like "ruler of the roost" as a child, threatening to have a tantrum unless his parents obeyed him. He also began to see how powerless he really had been and how his behavior protected him from this realization.

This material was difficult and painful for Mr. Lopez and for the therapist as they began to see even more clearly how ineffective his parents had been. In the following session Mr. Lopez began by saying, "I've been thinking about last time and my need for omnipotence—how I need to control situations. As a child I gave orders and even hit my mother. My parents couldn't control me." He continued to talk about a seductive, provocative mother who still talked with him about her sex life. He admitted to having sexual fantasies about her; sometimes they were violent. He wondered if the therapist could handle him. Maybe he'd want to kill her. More painful memories emerged and, after a period of rage and provocative behavior with the therapist, Mr. Lopez became sad and wanted to give up. Maybe he would kill himself. He blamed the therapist for his sadness. He was angry with himself for wanting a magic wand, hypnosis, an easy way out, and at the therapist for not giving him answers and easing his pain. Recalling what a tyrannical child he had been embarrassed and saddened him. The therapist explained how he had been hungry for consistent attention and boundaries and that his behavior had been an attempt to get his parents to give him these things.

In the ninth month of treatment Mr. Lopez reported having good thoughts about his once-hated probation officer. He was surprised at how much he appreciated this man who stood by him and helped him stay out of trouble. The therapist heard this as a transference message but filed it away. It was important for her to see a positive sign after sitting with and tolerating Mr. Lopez's tantrum-like behavior. Other positive signs took the form of some pleasant childhood memories. There had been a period in childhood when he was given gold stars for good hygiene. Another time his father gave him a dog. As these positive feelings about the past increased Mr. Lopez began blocking his thoughts about the therapist. He found it easier to keep her at a distance, avoiding his longings for closeness. In the past these hopes had been painfully dashed. Each time he trusted his parents he felt betrayed by their inability to love him consistently and appropriately. Eventually, he was able to express sadness and jealousy about the therapist's vacation. Realizing that she had an outside life was difficult for Mr. Lopez and he began sexualizing the transference rather than feeling his yearning for closeness. The therapist interpreted this defensive reaction and, although Mr. Lopez heard her, it became a repetitive theme over the many years of treatment.

In summary, I have tried to illustrate, using Mr. Lopez's first nine or ten months of treatment (which eventually shifted to analysis), how both patient and therapist tested each other and how the treatment deepened as trust was established. Techniques used in this initial phase of treatment included:

1. Listening with an ear to how the past affected the present;
2. Connecting actions outside of treatment to feelings about treatment and the therapist;
3. Forming diagnostic impressions with an eye to psychological-mindedness and ego strength;
4. Introducing the idea of free association;
5. Interpreting the patient's tendency to act rather than to feel and to articulate;

6. Introducing the concept of transference;
7. Setting limits and providing boundaries;
8. Permitting and interpreting regression in treatment;
9. Assessing the patient's resilience and the ability to tolerate therapeutic regression;
10. Listening for positive identifications as well as negative ones;
11. Evaluating the patient's ability to use interpretations of transference and resistance.

These technical measures were used with the list in Chapter 1 as backdrop. I do not mention listening for ego defect or deficit. Assessing the ego in these terms in order to determine the treatment plan can be imprecise and misleading especially in the first stage of treatment. Patients who have been severely damaged (see Miss Carter in Chapter 5) can do psychoanalytic work to varying degrees and should be given the opportunity to try. Therapists who look for developmental lags in determining what treatment is suitable run the risk of underestimating the patient's capabilities.

When uncomfortable issues threaten to reach consciousness or when the patient is faced with fresh anxiety she often doubts her capacity and the therapist's ability to handle the material or affect about to emerge. These doubts can be conscious, preconscious, or unconscious. The therapist detects the doubts and interprets them. Actions such as coming late, missing sessions, forgetting to pay, and threatening to quit treatment are some of the ways the patient tests the therapist. If the therapist maintains the frame and does not acquiesce to inappropriate requests or demands, choosing to explore the action instead, the patient is reassured that the therapist is comfortable and strong. This is not quite the same as analyzing resistance because resistance is ubiquitous and always present. Testing is viewed as a way to establish and reestablish trust.

To emphasize the purpose of deeper work I will review the concepts of transference and the tendency to repeat the past in the present. In doing psychoanalytic work the therapist allows herself to be a recipient of the patient's feelings, positive and negative and anything in between. Because patients (and people in general) perceive the present through lenses formed by past experience, the therapist is seen in ways that reflect past relationships and experiences, whether actual or fantasized. Echoes of the past affect how a person hears in the present. The tendency to repeat goes on in everyday life. The choices we make are always based to some degree and in some way on unconscious fantasies and perceptions of the past. Whereas people are chosen by the patient (and by people in general) and influenced to play set roles in an unconsciously scripted drama, the analyst's job is to comment on and to interpret the drama. Rather than react in kind to the patient's provocation, the therapist tries to weigh what transpires in a neutral, nonjudgmental, benevolently curious manner. I say "tries" because this is the most difficult part of our job and the crux of our work. To the degree that the therapist manages to interpret and not to get caught up in enacting with the patient, the work is useful. Enactment means that the patient and the therapist relive something together. This happens in all therapy, and is an important component in analytic work when spotted and understood.

> Mrs. Blue, an actress, was about to leave on tour. This entailed a five-week break in treatment. The therapist, after hearing anxiety in the material, suggested that Mrs. Blue might want to keep in touch regularly during her trip. At first Mrs. Blue responded positively. She had been brought up by self-involved parents who paid little attention to their children. The therapist's suggestion gratified a deeply felt need. However, before the trip Mrs. Blue decided that regular contact would be a step backward and would interfere with her hectic schedule. She said that she knew the therapist's phone number and would make use of it if necessary.

In reviewing the intervention, the therapist realized that she had imposed her wish to be helpful rather than letting the patient exercise her autonomy. The therapist overstepped her boundary by suggesting rather than interpreting. She had presumed to predict the patient's need based on her understanding and the patient's expression of anxiety, rather than remaining the neutral interpreter. She could have said something like, "I hear your anxiety about the separation. Have you any thoughts about how to handle it?" Why the therapist presumed to predict instead of remaining the neutral interpreter is an interesting question with many possible answers. She may have been responding to her own separation anxiety; she may have been nervous due to inexperience; she may have been responding to the patient's script as others had in the past; and she may have wished to avoid the patient's anger about the separation. Hindsight is helpful to the therapist because she can learn how to handle future dilemmas more effectively.

The therapist's job is to engage the patient in wondering about the patient's perception, behavior, and feelings, and, when appropriate, the therapist explains to the patient why she feels what she feels. But before such connections are attempted the therapist will let the patient's feelings become clear enough to identify by letting them intensify in the transference. How much the therapist waits depends on many factors such as:

1. The amount of time the patient has been in treatment;
2. The strength of the alliance;
3. The therapist's countertransference (e.g., is she bored, anxious, worried that the patient will leave?);
4. Is the patient coming frequently enough to contain the anxiety elicited by intense feelings?;
5. Diagnostic impressions (is the patient capable of hearing about the other person?);
6. The therapist's assessment of the patient's psychological mindedness and ability to reflect;
7. Is the patient threatening to disrupt the treatment?

The purpose of deepening the treatment is to permit new editions of old situations (sometimes called the *transference neurosis*) to emerge in the therapeutic setting so that patient and therapist can begin to understand such repetitions. The understanding is not merely intellectual, although the intellect is expanded; it is also emotional. The permission to express deep feelings heretofore repressed, split off, and avoided is not only cathartic. The expression of buried feelings reintroduces the patient to an important part of herself and frees the energy that had been spent denying those emotions expression.

The expression of feelings is also important in showing the patient that her feelings cannot destroy the hated object. Because buried feelings are often born in the patient's childhood omnipotent phase, the feelings are given enormous power in the unconscious. One of the difficulties in giving up the grandiose feelings is that the patient loses a sense of imagined power that has become gratifying. Also, the intense anger felt towards a parental figure, who has become intro-jected, is experienced as a threat to the self. The process takes vary-ing periods of time but it certainly takes a long time. When a person spends twenty years and more finding ways to defend against the anxiety produced by recognizing infantile wishes and fears, it is arro-gant and unrealistic of the therapist to be in any kind of hurry. The clinical reports of analysis being complete in three, four, or even five years set a standard that is false, in my experience. My experience comes from my own analysis, the analyses of colleagues who are open enough to share their experiences, from supervising people who seem to have had didactic rather than therapeutic analyses, and from my own work as an analyst.

Before reviewing the techniques on deepening the work let us look at what the patient is consciously and unconsciously thinking about. Consciously, there are issues of time and money but most frequently these issues mask the less conscious and unconscious fears every pa-tient experiences at different times during treatment.

"Can I do this?"
"How can she (the therapist) really be interested?"
"How will I know that she can understand me?"
"I know she'll think I'm awful if I tell all."
"I've never told these fantasies to anyone. Why would I tell her?"
"I've avoided closeness all my life. Why risk it now?"
"All she cares about is my money."
"If I face and express my rage I'll destroy us both."
"Is she strong enough to tolerate my rage?"

"I'll be so cooperative and interesting she'll fall in love with me."

"She'll seduce me or I'll seduce her. Then what?"

"I can manage my life now. Why risk the unknown?"

"Does she really know what she's doing?"

"I'll contaminate her."

"I'll drive her away with my needs and demands."

"I'll gain control the way I always do. I'll get her to change my appointment, not charge for sessions I miss, call me by my first name, pay late, not pay, threaten to quit if she doesn't play my way. Then I'll know she's afraid of me, or that all she wants is my money, or that she doesn't know what she's doing and that I am right not to trust her."

"I'll be so good, bring so many dreams, pay exactly on time, improve so much, she'll think I'm wonderful. I'll be her favorite patient and that will be enough for me. I'll finally be the star in someone's eyes. Then we can be friends forever. She'll really love me if I'm good."

"Once or twice a week will be enough. More would put her to sleep or bore her."

"Everyone I know goes once a week. Why should I need more? I must really be sick."

"I get great pleasure from my symptoms. My depression has become a friend. My masochistic behavior keeps me attached to the past. My guilt makes my suffering necessary."

"I'm afraid to go deeper. The water is safe here by the shore and I don't think I'll be safe out there. My feelings will drown me."

These quotes represent some possibilities of the conscious, preconscious, and unconscious thoughts a patient may have about change and trust.

Listening for the unconscious transference communications is the key to deepening the treatment. Once the patient begins to feel understood she is far more likely to trust the therapist. Hearing, understanding, and using the transference is the psychotherapist's most important tool in helping the treatment deepen. It is the patient's most important means of communication. Here is a vignette of a 28-

year-old man who sought therapy because he was feeling stuck in his life. He lived at home with his parents and held a job with potential for advancement. He had been in treatment once before and the therapist does not know why it ended. (It is helpful to find out about a patient's previous therapy experience in the consultation phase of treatment.) The focus will be on hearing the transference. Training the ear to hear this form of communication is necessary to hearing the unconscious.

Transference is ubiquitous. We all use our past experiences to formulate our present opinions and perceptions. A patient has transference fantasies and fantasies of cure before she makes the first phone call. As the treatment progresses these transference fantasies increase and when they stand in the way of going deeper they must be interpreted. This patient has been coming for one year.

Patient: Nothing's changed. I feel like I just try to get through each week. And you know, I fantasize so much every day and sometimes I wonder whether it gets in the way. But sometimes I think this is the closest I'm going to get. [laughs]

Therapist: The closest you'll get to what?

Patient: To succeeding. I guess I see that the fantasies aren't serving as an impetus to get me closer to anything.

Therapist: They're not serving as an impetus. Why might that be?

Patient: I'm afraid. And I don't feel that I have what it takes to really be on a certain level. You have to be someone who can be relied on to do a job and see it through to the end rather than run to someone for handholding. My boss just doesn't see me as someone who he can say "Here's the job—just get it done and send it out."

Therapist: What if he did see you that way?

Patient: Well, any euphoria I would feel would quickly be dampened by my fear about whether I could do the job.

Therapist: So there is ambivalence about whether or not you want to be seen this way.

Patient: Ambivalence? That just doesn't make sense to me. Why would I be ambivalent about this?

Therapist: Well, let's just say that there is a conflict about how you feel. Part of you wants to be thought of as someone who can be relied on and part of you doesn't.

Patient: You know, I think about people I see as players both socially and at work and I think about wanting to be part of that. You know, like a key player. People who are always looking for challenges. I hate to say it but I don't feel that's what I want. I wish that I wanted to be challenged but I'm too afraid of what could happen.

Therapist: And what could that be?

Patient: I might get in over my head. The worst scenario is that I would cause my firm to be sued by a major client—involving thousands of dollars in damages. [Later in the session the therapist makes a supportive remark about his functioning and the patient takes issue.]

Therapist: What just happened? I wonder if you were dampening my positive reaction.

Patient: Well, I feel that you're the doctor and I'm the patient and I have to make sure that you really understand in order for you to help me. If I say the problem is in my head and it's really in my foot, then you won't diagnose it properly.

Therapist: Hmm. Is there more to it?

Patient: You might think I'm fine and dismiss me.

This brief vignette, if looked at from a transference point of view, can tell us how the patient is feeling about therapy. He is telling his therapist that nothing has changed; that he has fantasies (about her) but worries that she doesn't want to hear them; that he's afraid that he "doesn't have what it takes" to succeed in treatment or with his therapist. He is afraid that he could do harm and cause much trouble if he asserted or expressed himself. He isn't sure he can be relied on to see this treatment through and he wonders if the therapist can be relied on. He worries that his therapist (boss) doesn't see him as someone who can see it through. (A previous treatment had ended.) He worries that the therapist will "dismiss" him. By saying this directly he is working with the transference feeling that his pain or fears will be overlooked.

How can the therapist be sure that the patient is talking about her and not just the boss? There is no proof. The patient is not necessarily aware that his comments are about his treatment and his therapist. It is the therapist's job to weigh the evidence that would indicate interpreting the transference meaning. The psychoanalytically oriented therapist learns that everything the patient brings into a session has transference meaning. Two people who meet regularly with no outside distraction will naturally develop thoughts and feelings about the other. In analytic work these thoughts and feelings become the major data. When and how the therapist uses the data of transference is based on skill that develops with experience. Earlier in the chapter I enumerated several factors that help determine when the material is ripe for interpretation. First we must learn to listen for transference manifestations. In the above vignette we may assume that because the therapist is usually perceived as the "boss" in the treatment, references to bosses in the patient's life often stand for the therapist. If this assumption is wrong the patient will reject it or correct it, but even if the patient rejects a linkage between therapist and boss it may still exist. Time will tell. The question is what might one do with this material to deepen the treatment by using the latent transference content. One thing to note is the first communication from the patient in each session, because the first comment is often a title to the hour. In this vignette "Nothing's changed" is the title. The patient then tells the therapist that he fantasizes every day and that he's afraid he hasn't got what it takes. How would we bring this material into the transference?

I would say something like, "While listening to what you've said I find myself wondering if your thoughts and feelings about work and your boss could also have to do with our work here and with me." If this was the first transference interpretation the patient might ask what I meant. I could then choose something in his material. For instance, I might say something like, "You began today saying that nothing was happening. Perhaps you feel that way about therapy," or "You said you fantasize every day. Can you tell me about your fantasies?" or "You expressed concern that I might think you're fine and dismiss you. Tell me about that."

These interventions are in the service of deepening the work. They let the patient know that the therapist is listening carefully and that she is willing to share her thoughts and to wonder. This process recording illustrates numbers 2, 8, and 9 in Chapter 1. The therapist has maintained her stance of benevolent curiosity in the face of her patient's passivity. He seems content to live with his parents and with his job level. However, he says that the therapy is his last hope and he shares a fantasy of destroying his firm and himself. The therapist feels distanced and ineffective at this point in treatment but she is aware that the patient is withholding important information. She knows very little about how the patient feels about her or about his early childhood and his relationship with parents and siblings. She lets the treatment unfold gradually by listening with respect and by being comfortable not knowing the answers or even the questions. As the patient gains trust he will begin to give hints of the deeper issues that bother him. We might speculate based on his fantasy of destroying the firm that he believes he has hidden power. We might imagine that he fears failure or that success is dangerous. (His uncle's failure in business was talked about in a previous session.) Nothing in the material or history (so far) indicates that this man could not do well with more intensive work. On the contrary, the patient seems frustrated with the twice-a-week sessions. His failure to continue treatment with a previous therapist, when explored, would help make this determination. His fantasy of destroying the firm can be heard in terms of the therapy.

The most important tool that the therapist has is the transference. Transference manifestations can be seen outside of treatment when, for example, a patient consistently sees authority figures as evil and unfair. If the therapist can hear this in terms of the therapy it is most helpful, but starting with the figures the patient presents comes first. For example, connecting the boss to an older, bossy sister who is in the material of the hour is a first step.

Hearing the patient's material in terms of her thoughts and feelings about the therapist is not difficult. Learning when to use what you hear requires experience and appropriate timing. By appropriate timing I mean keeping track of previous material and listening for when the patient is expressing affect.

Keeping track of the patient's references and obvious lack of references to the therapy and the therapist serves several purposes. For instance, if the patient suddenly notices something in the office that has been there all along, I hear this as a reference to the therapist. I do not necessarily interpret this but I think of what it might mean. Often this indicates that the patient feels safe enough to relate to me as a separate person. It usually means that the patient is feeling curious.

"Is that a new vase or picture?" "Is the plant new?" "I never noticed those books before." Such comments often indicate that the patient is interested in who the therapist is. This is a sign that the work is deepening.

Conversely, if the patient never mentions anything about the therapist or the therapy, avoids eye contact, and is often or suddenly silent the therapist can wonder what thoughts are occurring about her and what prevents the patient from speaking about them. In the beginning phase of therapy the therapist can explain that there will be thoughts and feelings about the therapist and that expressing these thoughts and feelings will be helpful to the work.

Encouraging and protecting the patient's curiosity and capacity for self-reflection can be accomplished without seeming intrusive by phrases such as:

What comes to mind about that?
I wonder if you have some more thoughts about that?
Do you suppose this has a connection to your dream?
Is that a familiar feeling?
Do you think that could have to do with missing your last session?
Can you elaborate?

These are gentle questions meant to help the patient reflect on the material. When the therapist is quite sure about hearing a connection there is no need to make the connection tentatively. Interpretations can be declarative statements and not just speculative invitations to entertain an idea.

Another important and sometimes overlooked technique in promoting self-reflection is silence. The sooner the therapist becomes comfortable being quiet the faster the treatment will deepen. Every intervention we make intrudes on the patient's thoughts. Interventions are important when made in a timely manner but often the therapist's need to be helpful or the pressure she feels to earn her fee makes her intervene prematurely. If we set the stage early in therapy by learning to be quiet the patient will feel free to see where her thoughts go. Being listened to quietly and nonjudgmentally is a new experience for most people, and although many therapists fear that their silence will frighten or displease the patient they quickly learn its value. This is also true when ending a session. "We'll stop for today" is all that's required in most instances. There is usually no need to wrap up a session for a patient.

If a patient lingers or continues to talk when the session is over there are different ways to respond.

> The therapist can repeat that it's time to stop and can invite the patient to continue the topic next time.
> The therapist can get up and walk to the door.
> The therapist can firmly say that there will be time to return to the subject.
> If the patient does not realize that the time is really up, the therapist can begin the next session by explaining why sessions are time-limited.
> The therapist can introduce the idea of more frequent sessions by saying something like, "You have much to say and once (or twice) a week doesn't seem like enough time. I think more frequent sessions would be valuable."

If the patient is ready to return to a topic in the next hour she will. If it is glaringly evident that she is avoiding what happened in the previous session the therapist can usually find something in the material that points out the avoidance, which is more useful than finding out what is avoided. Roy Schafer (1983) makes this point in his book *The Analytic Attitude*, where he describes how to analyze resistance before content. His example involves a patient who stifled her tears. Rather than wonder about what she wants to cry about he advocates addressing why she needs to stifle the crying.

Usually it is best to wait for the patient to return to a topic. If a topic is dropped the therapist can be sure that there is a reason. Letting things unfold involves letting the patient determine what she wants to say and what she wants to avoid, consciously or unconsciously. If the patient says, "I can't remember what happened last time," this can be a clue to wanting more time. It can also mean "Do you remember my last session?" The therapist can encourage the patient to explore the possible meanings of her question or statement.

Some patients prefer or can't help staying very close to the surface. They are used to thinking in very concrete terms and seem to be unable even to wonder if there is more than what meets the eye.

Mr. Green was such a person. He came to treatment on the advice of his friend who was in analysis with a colleague. He was in turmoil about the demands his mistress was putting on him. He was a married man and the idea of ending his 30-year marriage was unthinkable, yet he was forced to consider it because his lover was putting pressure on him to decide between her and his wife. Mr. Green found it impossible to focus on anything but his real and present problem, and the therapist could only wait for things to unfold. It emerged that Mr. Green's only daughter was to be married in a month and as he talked about the upcoming wedding his emotions surfaced. There was also sadness about his aging parents, who were getting frail and unable to care for themselves. Talking about these events and feelings calmed Mr. Green and he reported that his high blood pressure decreased. He learned that his initial and presenting problem was covering other painful feelings that no one had heard—including himself. He was amazed at his depth of feeling. One day I asked Mr. Green if he remembered his dreams. He said no, but after a few weeks he began to remember dream fragments. It could be said that he was trying to please me, but that was interpretable and the dreams gave him a new part of himself to work with. Mr. Green became increasingly comfortable with my listening stance. It freed him to see where his thoughts led, and the treatment deepened as a result.

What happens when the treatment doesn't deepen? What are the consequences of passing up opportunities to examine and understand with the patient the roadblocks that are inevitable in psychotherapy? In this book I discuss the patient's right to test the waters and to travel at her own pace. The therapist has the duty, however, to listen for opportunities to deepen the work. Walking the fine line between not pushing a patient and remembering that connecting past and present depends upon in-depth work requires skill, timing, and most of all the conviction that second chances become possible by looking inside. Patients test the therapist at different times during treatment while developing the trust necessary to making the commitment to ongoing, intensive work. The following vignette can be looked at with this in mind.

Mrs. Hawkins, toward the end of her fourth year in treatment, announced that she was seriously contemplating taking a month off from therapy in order to save money. She told her therapist, Dr. S., that although she was giving only two days notice, she really hoped Dr. S. would understand and not be angry, the way her former therapist had been when she did the same thing. She jokingly said that Dr. S. would probably kick up her heels during the break. Mrs. Hawkins seemed determined to act on her plan. She asked Dr. S. if she could feel free to call during the break if she needed an appointment. Dr. S. felt helpless in the face of this "fait accompli" and her efforts to explore the action proved fruitless. She even offered to defer the fee until Mrs. Hawkins felt less financially strapped. Mrs. Hawkins remained adamant.

When a patient *contemplates* taking action, even when short notice is given, the therapist can say something like: "While I understand your situation logically I think it would be important to explore other, less conscious motivations before you act. Can you see what comes to mind?" or "You mention that you're contemplating taking time off. That sounds like you haven't decided definitely. Can you talk about the pros and cons of the action?" These comments and others like them tell the patient that you are concerned, unafraid, and dedicated to preserving the rhythm of the work. Mrs. Hawkins had shared the fantasy that the therapist would "kick up her heels" during the break. Was she worried that the work was becoming too heavy or boring? This fantasy would be important to explore. The therapist might say something like: "It sounds as though you think I would be delighted to have a break. Tell me about that."

When Mrs. Hawkins returned after the month off she was in high spirits.

Patient: I have so much to say—some good things and other harder things. I started three paintings during the month. It feels terrific. Annie walks to school by herself now so I don't have that *commitment which is death to me.* (More details about the month off; pause) Now I have to talk about the not so happy thoughts or the hard thoughts. I want to talk but how can I tell you? *Just because I say it—it doesn't mean I have to act on it. Nothing has to happen, it's all right to talk about it—those are your words I hear in my head.* I absolutely loved the freedom this month. Not coming here freed up two days. I had no decisions about when to work or when to paint. I don't have to feel all that horrible telling you. *I know I don't make you furious at me—at least when I'm here in the room.*

Therapist: Not in the room? What about that?

Patient: (ignores question) I felt *I was out of school*—like summer vacation when *you let me take an extra month off and don't charge me so I have two months away.* The closer I got to coming back the more conflicted I felt. I had a great month. Not that I don't need therapy. Was the month easy because I didn't have to come here and think about things? *Maybe keeping a lid on things is why I did so well. Is there a fear of some unknown thing that I know deep down I have to talk about?* Having the extra

> money was great. *The thought of coming in here and it being my last day is so frightening and so sad. My fantasy is that once I walk out, that's it.* Then in six months—do I dare say it? I guess I could start up if you were available. *Don't worry, I'm not planning any escape tomorrow.* Also, I know I can take you with me!

What is Mrs. Hawkins saying beneath the manifest content? The italicized phrases or remarks are important to explore and to understand.

1. *Commitment is like death.* Patient tells how frightened she is.
2. *Nothing has to happen.* Patient reassures therapist.
3. *I don't have to act—I can talk. You taught me that.* Patient says she has gained something from therapy.
4. *Do I make you furious at me?* Patient is worried that therapist will lose patience and wonders if she can provoke the therapist to be angry. When therapist tries to explore patient's thoughts about being furious *at least not in the room* patient ignores her. (When a patient ignores a therapist's intervention this can be pointed out with an interested, benignly curious tone by a comment like: "I noticed that you seem to want to avoid my question. What comes to mind?" If the therapist lets a comment about anger go, she runs the risk of letting the patient think that anger is to be avoided.)
5. *You let me go for two months in the summer.* Patient has thoughts and feelings about the long separation and the fact that therapist does not charge her, thereby sanctioning it.
6. References to *being out of school* and *escaping* tell therapist that she is seen as an authority figure.
7. *I'm afraid of some unknown thing deep down.* Patient asks therapist if she is afraid too.
8. *The thought of my last day is frightening and sad.* Patient is saying "don't let me go."

Dr. S. was being given another chance at deciphering the action, this time before it occurred. It is important to explain that when Mrs. Hawkins began treatment, Dr. S. was beginning her private practice and her training. Like many beginning therapists she had not felt confident enough to state a policy about charging for extra vacations. In a supervisory consultation following the first session after the break Dr. S. examined her countertransference. She felt as if her hands had been tied. Fearful of losing her patient she felt she could have done nothing to prevent the month break in treatment. At first she thought of the break as a rapprochement enactment with the patient attempting to go out into the world and come back to safety like a young child does with her mother. She also had feelings about being "laid off" for a month. After reviewing the sessions in supervision she began to consider the action as a test and a provocation. The patient seemed to be saying several things. "Are you afraid of my anger?" "Can I overpower you and control you as I have felt controlled?" "Do you really want to hear about the unknown things I keep deep inside?" "I'll show you how sudden abandonment feels." "You'll be happy to have a rest from me. You let me go for an extra month in the summer and maybe you're so relieved to be rid of me that you don't charge as you do for other missed sessions."

Dr. S. decided that more activity on her part was necessary when faced with Mrs. Hawkins's thoughts about ending treatment. This does not mean that she could prohibit her patient from action but that she would maintain her attitude of benevolent curiosity to find out what lay beneath the proposed action. Remembering that the patient hires the therapist and always has the final word helps the therapist avoid tiptoeing. If the therapist does her work chances are that the patient will feel encouraged to do *her* work.

Dr. S. could say something like: "I understand the reality of your wish but can you put that aside for a while and see what comes to mind?" "I wonder if something here in the treatment is making you want to retreat." "You mentioned the extra month you take off in the summer and that I allow that. Talk about how it feels to have such a long break." "If you can put your feelings into words we can begin to understand why you feel you need a break." "It seems that this idea to end therapy has a component of anger that may be easier to put into action than express in words." "Perhaps you worry that I need a rest. What does that mean?" "Talk about your fantasy of me kicking my heels up."

The supervisor also encouraged Dr. S. to state her present policy about missed sessions by saying something like: "I know that in the past I have not charged you for missed vacation sessions but my policy has changed. Because your appointments belong to you, when you're not here I cannot fill them. Most important I think that breaks, aside from a month vacation in summer and a few weeks during the winter (if that is her policy), jeopardize our work seriously because we lose continuity." Said in a calm, firm, concerned manner, this intervention is meant to deepen the treatment. The therapist is saying: "I care about our time together. I can tolerate your feelings and I am not bored with or frightened of our work. I can take care of myself. It is safe to express your feelings in here. You may be concerned about the unknown but I'm confident that we can face your fears together. Burying them is not the answer."

Dr. S. also began to see the sadomasochistic aspect of her patient's taking a month off. She filed this away because she felt she needed more evidence but she did introduce the idea that Mrs. Hawkins was angry. Whenever there is a separation between patient and therapist (Chapter 6) there is anger that must be explored in words.

I have tried to illustrate through this vignette that after four years of important work the patient started to balk. Her action alerted the therapist that she was frightened of going deeper. The therapist then took the opportunity to work with her patient on understanding and interpreting so that the treatment could deepen.

An interesting dilemma occurs when a patient comes in crisis and states that she can only be in treatment for a limited time. Crisis intervention is a specialty in the field of psychotherapy but here crisis will be looked at in psychoanalytic terms. When a crisis is brought on by the patient we must look at it as a communication.

A colleague consulted about a young man who came to her after an accident he had at college that required surgery. The patient was traumatized by the accident. As a result of the accident the patient was unable to complete his semester. He was due to leave for Europe in six months in order to spend his junior year abroad. My colleague felt pressured to accomplish something with this young man but she was perplexed as to how much she could deepen the work. Because she identified herself as an analyst I felt that this was how she must approach the material.

In the first session with the patient (who will be referred to as Mr. A.) the therapist learned a great deal. What was most important, she felt, was his awareness that he had been depressed ever since he could remember, that he drank alcohol every day, and that he was not "so drunk" the night of the accident. He also told the therapist that he had been having "negative thoughts" for several months. When asked to tell about the thoughts he said that he couldn't stand the pressure anymore, that he had packed a bag many months ago, went to the highway to hitchhike and run away, but was frightened by thoughts of jumping in front of a car. In addition the therapist saw that Mr. A. had all the vegetative symptoms of a major depression. She told him that medication was indicated and that she wanted to see him as many times a week as possible. She also shared with him that his accident was an unconscious attempt to get out of an intolerable situation. Mr. A. asked, "Can the unconscious do that?" My colleague told him that the unconscious was very powerful and that they could learn more in their sessions.

During the next two sessions Mr. A. described other suicidal gestures such as practicing unsafe sex and using various dangerous drugs. In the fourth session he asked the therapist if he should go to Europe. The therapist said that they would decide together as they learned more.

This vignette illustrates several things:

1. The therapist's initial response of pressure was a countertransference response to the patient's feeling pressured.
2. The therapist used her analytic background, with its respect for the unconscious, in order to understand this young man.
3. The therapist respected the patient's autonomy by not giving advice but instead by inviting him to join her in deciding what was best.
4. Had the therapist advised the patient to cancel his plans she would have stepped out of her neutral position. Although

she felt that the trip was ill-advised, she avoided a possible power struggle by offering to collaborate with the patient in the decision.

5. The therapist referred the patient for medication to alleviate the depression. This decision was based on Mr. A.'s symptoms.

Another way of handling the question would have been saying to the patient something like, "From what you've told me it sounds like you have ambivalent or mixed feelings about the trip and serious concerns about the way you feel in general. I think these concerns can be best understood in psychotherapy." Hearing the therapist's impression under serious circumstances such as this can be relieving to a troubled patient. In this case the patient's parents were interested only in his performance and unable to adjust their expectations for their son, even when informed of the son's self-destructive behavior and depression. This was the pressure felt by both therapist and patient. When faced with suicidal behavior and major depression the therapist owes it to the patient to express concern and to offer a course of action. In this case the therapist did recommend medication and indicated to the patient that they would decide about future plans together.

I can't end this chapter without mentioning the patient who talks nonstop, never seeming to pause for air. Session after session goes by and the therapist literally can't get a word in edgewise. Such nonstop talking must be seen as a message. Some call it a resistance, which it certainly is; labeling it a resistance takes us only so far, though. The therapist, along with feeling assaulted, attacked, or shut out, uses her benevolent curiosity. This is the best safeguard against letting countertransference rule the day.

Miss Gilbert chattered incessantly and annoyingly during her sessions. Mr. D., her therapist, presented this dilemma in class. He was beyond feeling curious and was indeed furious at his patient. Members of the class commiserated and then tried to help him regain the feeling that he was indeed the therapist and not the victim. (Being in a class, seminar, or supervision group when treating patients is invaluable in maintaining a therapeutic perspective.) The class pointed out that the incessant talking was both defensive and aggressive. The class reminded him that at some point he would find a place to intervene *if* he could regain his neutral, interested stance. The point was made that Mr. D.'s distress and anger were registering with the patient in subtle and some not so subtle ways. (He forgot one appointment and was late for several others.) Once he regained his curious attitude the class felt that Mr. D. would find a way and a place to say something.

Here are some of the things he might say:

"If my therapist kept me waiting for an appointment I'm sure I'd have some feelings. Will you tell me yours?"
"I wonder if you're worried that I might say something upsetting because it seems hard for me to find a place to say anything."
"Have you noticed that I never say anything?"
"Sometimes I wonder if beneath all the things you say are feelings you'd rather not deal with."
"I worry that you want to keep me out. Is it because you fear I'll say something hurtful?"

If there is something in the patient's material that would shed light on her need to shut the therapist out this might give the therapist a clue. Miss G. did speak of an intrusive, meddlesome mother, and the therapist might say something like, "Perhaps you worry that I will be intrusive and bossy, too." All of the above suggestions are naturally meant to deepen the work by engaging the patient in benevolent curiosity.

In a well-conducted psychotherapy, after a period of testing, there will often be signals that the patient is ready to deepen the treatment in terms of frequency. What are the cues? A patient might say:

"The session went by so quickly."
"There never seems to be enough time."
"I hope I remember this dream until we meet again."
"I thought about calling you after our last session."

"Why do people use the couch?"
"I can't remember what we talked about last time."

Actions can convey the wish for deeper work:

Coming early for appointments;
Looking at the couch frequently;
Telephoning between sessions;
Putting one's jacket or other belongings on the couch;
Leaning back in the chair and looking away from the therapist;
Requesting extra sessions;
Coming on the wrong day.

How the therapist responds to these signals or cues can determine the future course of the work. With tact and appropriate timing the treatment should deepen quite naturally.

❖ CHAPTER 4 ❖

Considering the Patient's Pace— How Often Is Often Enough?

Although psychoanalytic work is best done from two to five times a week, many patients cannot commit to this optimal frequency at the start. The reasons for frequent sessions include: establishing continuity, providing conditions for the recognition and working through of transference phenomena, setting up conditions for consistent work, containing anxiety, and providing support.

Continuity is necessary in any learning endeavor, whether it be studying a new language (like the unconscious), a new sport, or a musical instrument. The process of looking inside is new to many people who come to the analytically oriented therapist. Being listened to nonjudgmentally and with benevolent curiosity with the aim of understanding is a new experience for most patients. Frequent sessions enable the therapeutic dyad to connect material from session to session more easily and convincingly.

Transference is ubiquitous. Every patient and every therapist develop transferences to each other from the very first contact. In fact, before the patient makes her first appointment she has expectations and fantasies based on her past about treatment and about the therapist. Transference is a most valuable tool in psychoanalytic work because it shows us how the past resonates in the present. The psychoanalytically oriented therapist makes use of transference manifestations in order to help the patient understand why and how the past lives in the present. The more often a patient can come to treatment, the clearer the transference picture becomes. In fact, it is negative transference (negative expectations) that often inhibits a patient from trusting the therapist enough to come more often. Patients who have been disappointed early in life expect more of the same, and it often takes years before they can begin to trust. This is why a "wading in" approach must be considered.

Consistency means reliability, which many patients have never experienced. Patients test the therapist in many ways to determine just how reliable she is by missing appointments, asking to reschedule appointments, wanting to cut down or end therapy, and coming very early or very late to see if the therapist will alter the agreed-upon time. Reliability and consistency are crucial to the development of trust, so it is important for the patient to see the therapist maintain her neutral, inquiring, nonretaliatory stance. Anxiety arising because of transference fantasies, wishes, and fears can be allayed by frequent sessions.

Support is not often mentioned as a psychoanalytic technique because the psychoanalytically oriented therapist does not take sides. However, being listened to with benevolent curiosity and respect is unique; protecting and fostering a patient's autonomy is supportive in the very deepest sense. When a patient has had a traumatic past where her individuality has not been cherished, her hope for a second chance lies with someone who will not repeat past "sins." Patients who use sadomasochistic solutions to preserve ties to past objects need years of intensive work so that new identifications can replace and soften old ones.

This chapter is about how to listen for and interpret patients' conflicts about increasing sessions and going deeper.

Miss Donavan, an intelligent, articulate 21-year-old, came to a clinic in a state of depression with thoughts of suicide. She lived at home with her alcoholic mother and four siblings. The home was chaotic and in a state of disrepair. Miss Donavan worked and attended college at night. She spent most of her free time with her boyfriend, Ray, who was kind, caring, and supportive and held a steady job. The two had been dating since high school and their relationship was serious.

In the beginning of her second year of once-a-week therapy Miss Donavan mentioned having thoughts of suicide. The therapist who had brought up increasing the number of sessions several months prior brought it up again, but Miss Donavan said she couldn't afford it. The therapist felt she could not insist.

The following excerpt is from her 55th session:

Patient: (walks in, five minutes late, with head down, making no eye contact) I'm so down today, I just couldn't get up. I woke up on time but I couldn't get going. I've been like this all weekend. The semester is almost over and I don't want to do the work. I've been procrastinating about a lot of things like going to the eye doctor. (talks about insurance paperwork) I've got to just go ahead and get this taken care of. I'm getting headaches and I know it's from eyestrain.

Therapist: What do you think this is about?

Patient: Well, I was supposed to go out with my friend Carol on Friday to celebrate my promotion—we had made definite plans and she canceled. She was hemming and hawing about not being sure. We've been planning this for ages. So when Ray called I told him and he said he would take me out to the movies. It was great fun. I wanted to go again on Saturday but he had a basketball game. I needed to study on Saturday anyway, but I didn't. I procrastinate all the time. I keep putting things off. I watched TV instead of working on my paper for school. I could have done it at Ray's house because he has room for me to study—but I didn't. I don't know why.

Therapist: Your low mood and difficulty getting going this morning— is this all related to your disappointment for not getting your paper done over the weekend?

Patient: I think so. I was like this yesterday, too. Running late for work because I overslept. Then I forgot my wallet and had to go back home to get it. It was Valentine's Day and Ray took me to a lovely restaurant. He brought flowers and a beautiful bracelet. He said he loves me. After dinner I twisted my ankle and was hobbling around like my mother, who walks a few steps and then has to stop to catch her breath. When I got home my mother was drunk and didn't even say hello. I'm working so hard in school and she never asks about how I'm doing or what I'm doing. I don't have any support from her—I wish she was

there for me. I need more encouragement, more support. Ray
tries so hard. He gave me a Precious Moments statue. I love
Precious Moments—I collect them and I have a few.

What is Miss Donavan telling her therapist in terms of transference? What is beneath her conscious communication? What is the latent content? *I am so disappointed that I can't get up in the morning. The year here is almost over and I don't want to do this work. I don't know why and I'm not sure you really know because you don't tell me. I put off taking care of myself. You offered to see me more often but I need more encouragement. You have a place for me to study myself and I can't use it. I don't know why. I get in my own way and procrastinate. Like Ray, you try, but it's not enough. He gave me Precious Moments, which is what I need here. At least I can identify with my mother who limps through life. Better to be like her than risk change.*

It is now the therapist's job to find appropriate and timely ways to translate these latent messages to her patient. She could begin by saying something like, "You tell me how very disappointed you are in your mother and in yourself and how you need encouragement and support to do the hard work that needs to be done. I think you are disappointed in me, too. I want to remind you that I can see you more often and that more moments here will be precious. Aside from the extra $20 a week, what comes to mind about seeing me more often?"

When the therapist sees that a patient is in intense pain, talking of suicide and having physical symptoms, it is her obligation to focus on the obstacles to more frequent sessions. Miss Donavan's history and her present life cause her great pain. It seems that clinging to the pain is part of her neurosis. In order to extricate herself she needs more help than once a week can offer. In fact, once a week can be seen as yet another frustration to which she clings.

In this case the therapist has considered her patient's pace and sees that it is not appropriate to the situation. It is her job to engage her patient in quickening it. She has begun that process by arranging for a second session. Now she can listen for what stops her patient.

Mr. Steele, age 38, lived with his abusive wife and two children. He began therapy because he was depressed and had thoughts of suicide. Life at home was miserable and his wife refused marriage counseling. He was worried about the effect his wife's drinking and verbal abuse would have on his children, yet he seemed paralyzed and unable to do anything about this long-standing situation. A friend referred him to Dr. R., who came to consult with me. Dr. R. knew that once a week would not be enough and told his patient that he would benefit by coming more often, and yet his patient refused. Here is a vignette from the sixth month of treatment.

Patient: I could hardly get here today. I missed work yesterday—just stayed home and watched TV until the kids came home. I'm not much company to them but at least I'm there. Laura is away on business this week. Maybe there's another man. This has happened before but it gets harder and harder to take. She'll be back and be remorseful for a few days. She'll cut down on the drinking for a while—but she'll start again.

Therapist: You're in a lot of pain.

Patient: It's been worse. Another problem is work. Don (boss) promised me a raise months ago but never came through. I'm afraid to push it but it's so frustrating. On top of all this I had a minor car accident this morning. I had one of my headaches and I just lost my concentration for a minute and stopped too short for the light. Someone rear-ended me. No one got hurt but it scared me. I can't trust myself. Maybe Laura is right to be fed up with me. Maybe I'm just a loser. My brother and his wife side with me. They keep telling me to leave her and have even offered to let me and the kids stay with them.

Therapist: How did that offer feel?

Patient: Well, they have a huge place but I can't imagine them really wanting us. They have kids and jobs and—I don't know—maybe they really mean it. My brother has always looked out for me. When I was a kid he'd intercede with my father for me. Dad was a rigid guy and could be pretty abusive.

> *Therapist:* You hardly ever talk about your childhood.
>
> *Patient:* What does that have to do with anything? I have enough problems today without dredging all that up.
>
> *Therapist:* Things that happen in childhood have a way of coloring the present.

What is Mr. Steele saying to his therapist beneath the manifest level? *I'm really depressed. I'm disappointed. My brother (therapist) offers help but I can't trust that he (you) means it. I'm afraid I'll hurt myself (car accident) and I don't know what to do. My father hurt me as a kid and there's nothing I can do about that. You offer to see me more often but I'm a loser and you'll get tired of me. The past is painful and I'm afraid to look at it.*

What can Dr. R. say to his patient based on this material? *"I hear your despair and your concern. I think that you may be disappointed in me, too. I suggested that you increase your sessions and I never brought it up again. You may be afraid that if you let me know you better, I'll judge you as your wife does and as your father did. What comes to mind about seeing me more often?"*

Patients who come to a therapist knowing little about the process usually need to test the process and the therapist.

Mr. Taylor had a history of abuse. His father was moody and unpredictable, resorting to physical punishment at times. After the sixth month of psychoanalytic work he was torn between the wish to go deeper by increasing his sessions and the fear of facing the painful feelings that he had hidden for so many years. The following vignette illustrates his fear of trusting the analyst.

> *Patient:* I didn't feel like being here today. Things are going well in my life and I can't seem to justify paying all this money. I keep dreaming of money and can't decide if I can afford to come more often or not. Are you saying that if I don't add a session this will be a mistake?
>
> *Therapist:* I can't say that. I can only try to help you see what frightens you. Then you'll be better able to decide.

Patient: (long silence)

Therapist: Where did you go?

Patient: I was looking at all those books you have. I can't believe you've read them all. Maybe you read between patients but I doubt it. I see a book I'm familiar with. It used to be a favorite. *Call It Sleep* by Henry Roth. I can't remember what it was about but it was wonderfully written. I had it in paperback and when it got yellow with age I threw it away. No sense in keeping old books.

Therapist: The book was about a boy who was abused by his father. I think you're telling us how you've tried to throw away those feelings about your father. Coming here more often threatens to revive them.

Patient: I guess you're right. I had no memory of the book being about abuse. But I still can't understand how digging all that up will help me. My problem these days is whether to get engaged to Lois. She's putting pressure on me and I keep balking.

Therapist: It's hard for you to let yourself feel close to Lois—and to me, too. Closeness threatens you with pain and disappointment.

Patient: I don't think I'll ever let anyone really close to me. It's better this way. But I do love Lois and I want marriage and a family. If I get into this analysis will my fears go away?

Therapist: I think what will happen is that you'll be able to put these fears in perspective. The disappointment and pain go back to when you were little. You've covered them up pretty successfully but you haven't been able to throw them away like you did with the book. They still affect you.

Patient: How can I know it's safe to do that? I'm not sure I even like you. Why do you keep all of these books and why isn't your office nicer? This chair is so old and the couch looks so uncomfortable.

Therapist: It feels safer to keep me at a distance by disapproving of me.

Patient: I can see that—what difference does it make about your office. But maybe it does make a difference. Maybe you're depressed or poor. Maybe you just need my money. I can twist things any-

> way I want to—I can also see that you're smart and that you
> seem calm and that you do seem to understand me so far.

In this vignette the analyst maintains his neutral stance by not taking sides for or against increasing sessions, but tries instead to make
the patient aware of the fears that stand in his way of deepening the
work.

As helpful as frequent sessions are, it is important that the patient choose to increase sessions when she feels ready. The therapist can avoid making this issue a power struggle by listening to the
material for signs of the patient's conflicts and ambivalence about
deepening the work and pointing them out, using tact and appropriate timing. The following case illustrates that important work can
be done once a week and that it can take many years for a patient
to increase the frequency of sessions. Analyzing resistance does not
always work and must sometimes take a back seat to respecting the
patient's pace.

Dr. G. came for consultation about Mr. Irving whose youngest child
was dying of leukemia. The patient could only commit to weekly sessions. During the second year of therapy Mr. Irving's son died and a
long period of mourning followed. In the early years of a long treatment Mr. Irving told his story. He was a Holocaust survivor, having
escaped from Germany with his parents when he was 5 years old. He
spent the next ten years in Denmark, and then came to the United
States to rejoin his relatives. He had developed a stoic attitude towards
life and found it very hard to face, on an emotional level, the difficulties
he experienced in his childhood. After many years in treatment he slowly
and gradually began to look beneath his defensive denial and avoidance. He realized that how he related to his wife and to his therapist
deprived him of feeling close. He saw that his distancing mechanisms
protected him from future loss while making him feel lonely and deprived in the present. In therapy he dealt with his anger, fear, and
despair every week. The analyst felt strongly that his patient could benefit
from more frequent sessions but Mr. Irving would not consider the

idea. Dr. G.'s acceptance had a profound impact on his patient, who had never before been consulted about his needs or wishes. Is this an analytic technique? Should the therapist not analyze Mr. Irving's resistance instead of accepting his position? Was this an "enactment resistance" described by Rothstein (1990, p. 154) meant to frustrate the therapist? I would see the refusal to increase sessions as based on fear of closeness and anxiety about reliving extremely painful emotions. Mr. Irving's life experience as a survivor and as a parent who lost a child were factors that had to be weighed in terms of the pain involved in intensive psychoanalytic work.

Private space and time to himself were precious to Mr. Irving. He valued them above everything. His job and his family were responsibilities he could not ignore. Coming to therapy was important but his therapist's ability to value his time and space turned out to be of crucial importance. Analysis of this stance as a resistance proved useless. Mr. Irving's reluctance to expose the fear and pain of his childhood and his preference for stoicism were explored, but it was the therapist's acceptance of Mr. Irving's decision and his respect for Mr. Irving's autonomous functioning that permitted the treatment to deepen. Dr. G. was a trained analyst. He listened and thought analytically. He interpreted resistance and transference manifestations and he encouraged free association. He did not give advice nor did he share personal information. He engaged Mr. Irving in seeing how the past affected the present. Both patient and analyst made reconstructions and interpretations. The couch was not used and frequency did not qualify the treatment as psychoanalysis but Dr. G. and I felt that psychoanalytic work was done. In his sixth year of treatment Mr. Irving decided to increase his sessions to twice a week. The painful mourning period was as complete as it could be and his relationship with his wife had become increasingly difficult. Dr. G. brought up a second session again and, because it made sense, Mr. Irving agreed. Dr. G. and I felt that this was due to the completion of mourning, the ego strengthening that had taken place, and the trust in the analyst and in his method. Mr. Irving felt enough trust to begin exploring his need to keep his therapist on a pedestal. Past anger was slowly directed to the therapist in the transference and Mr. Irving's masochistic tendencies slowly began to shift as he directed this anger away from himself.

Mr. Haft began treatment on the insistence of his third wife. The referral was accepted reluctantly and the patient was not willing or motivated to come more than once a week.

Mr. Haft's father was a diplomat who traveled frequently with his wife. Neither parent had time for the five children, who were brought up by servants. The family moved frequently to different countries and, although the children attended American schools, making friends was difficult and seemed futile. Mr. Haft's face was scarred from a burn he suffered while playing with matches when he was 6. He had been left unattended and was rushed to the hospital by a chauffeur. Both parents were out of the country and returned several days after his hospitalization. Mr. Haft remembered a lonely childhood with minimal attention from adults. His father took him on a trip once when he was 4 and this exclusive attention meant everything to him. His oldest sister favored him and taught him to play tennis and ride horses. When he spoke of such memories he cried and was surprised by his strong emotions.

Relating these incidents along with present life problems was the focus of the first year's sessions. Mr. Haft continued to be skeptical about therapy. It was usually difficult for him to want to come to his weekly sessions and he canceled appointments frequently. The therapist told him that he would find it easier if he increased to twice a week. When he realized that it was hard for him to leave sessions and that he did want more time he agreed to twice a week but his resistance continued. Many sessions were canceled at the last minute and sometimes he did not call at all. The therapist waited. Once he came one minute before his time was up and saw Dr. F. waiting. These cancellations were a test. Would the therapist lose patience or interest? Was she really reliable? Mr. Haft paid for his many missed appointments without complaint. He expected to be charged. Later he admitted that due to his provocation it had been hard for him to believe the professional atmosphere would last. Sometimes, while waiting for Mr. Haft the therapist felt annoyed and hopeless. In supervision, I encouraged her to wait. A vacation exacerbated the situation. Mr. Haft missed sessions before and after the one-week vacation, saying he had misunderstood when the therapist would return. The therapist did in fact call Mr. Haft after his second missed appointment and he returned to treatment.

Dr. F. told Mr. Haft that she would not charge him for the sessions he thought she had canceled while at the same time she explained that the misunderstanding might have been caused by Mr. Haft's anger or other feelings about the vacation. This was difficult for him to acknowledge but he did associate to his son's negative reaction to separation. Using Mr. Haft's son to understand how a 3-year-old feels and expresses his feelings was a very useful technique. Mr. Haft saw how attention and lack of attention affected his child and he began to understand how much he had buried his feelings about neglect.

Memories of deprivation and loneliness emerged. Many times during this remembering Dr. F. pointed out that Mr. Haft was smiling. It became clearer that Mr. Haft defended against sadness and despair with a smiling, stoic attitude. Presenting this defensive posture and connecting it to its purpose—avoidance of pain—allowed Mr. Haft to begin to face these feelings with empathy and respect. He had never felt permission, from himself or others, to cry and doing so became safe.

This initial work with Mr. Haft was made possible by Dr. F.'s patience, consistency, and respect. Techniques of explanation, reconstruction, and education (by learning from children's reactions and behaviors) helped Mr. Haft deepen the treatment. At no time did the therapist change her analytic posture or manipulate the frame. Mr. Haft's major difficulty in life was his procrastination. In order to modify this character trait psychoanalysis was the treatment of choice. His need and ability to test the waters was respected and he became convinced when Dr. F. passed his tests. Because of his compliant façade he may have agreed to begin analysis at the start but Dr. F. was able to permit him to choose for himself.

In the second year of treatment Mr. Haft reported the sudden wish to have an affair with a colleague he had met for lunch that day. He found this distressing and confusing. His therapist brought the wish into the transference by reminding her patient that he had been considering adding a session two months ago and the subject had been dropped. She asked him if he thought this had to do with his wish for an affair. Mr. Haft's responded, "Suddenly I have a feeling of warmth. The shawl near your chair is like a blanket and I can imagine curling up on the couch with a cup of tea. I guess I really do want more time here."

Mr. Haft's ability to translate his temptation to act out his wish for closeness with the colleague into words impressed him and the therapist. The treatment had deepened.

There is a very fine line between the therapist's wish to give the patient the best possible treatment and the patient's option to choose based on her own readiness for and conviction about the process. I submit that, as convinced as the analyst is about the benefits of analysis, it must make sense to the patient. It must also feel as safe as it can, notwithstanding the natural anxiety inherent in looking inside. By viewing a patient's reluctance as pure resistance the analyst risks creating a power struggle. Such a stance makes it seem as though the analyst is serving her own needs and wishes. Indeed, Rothstein (1995) admits that it makes him and his colleagues feel better thinking of themselves as conducting analysis. This bias or preference diminishes the importance of well-conducted psychoanalytic psychotherapy that often leads to the deepest work of analysis. Designating the beginning phase of therapy as either preparation for analysis, trial analysis or analysis seems to put an unnecessary label on a naturally unfolding process. There may be no harm in this but it can lead to a pressure on the analyst to make things happen that happen naturally: deepening the work. I have found that, if permitted, a set of transferences evolve naturally. When these transference manifestations are identified and explored, patient and therapist begin to understand how perceptions are affected by the past. Such understanding in itself makes certain defenses unnecessary. Consistent interpretation of how a rigid and inhibiting character style preserves a status quo and learning why the status quo is hard to relinquish is what analysis is all about.

How a person chooses this long-term form of treatment should depend on her ability and right to test the waters. If the therapist proves to be a respectful, capable, trustworthy guide and the psycho-analytic journey makes sense, the two parties will embark.

In Mr. Haft's case his therapist's ability to be respectful, consistent, and benevolently curious engaged him in a process he had never considered: seeing how the past affects the present. His self-criticism and shame diminished gradually as he internalized his therapist's stance, and this process led to deeper work.

During Dr. W.'s supervision with me he talked about Ms. Pratt whom he had been seeing twice a week for many years. His work with this 40-year-old guarded woman had been frustrating and perplexing because although she canceled frequently and regularly she had maintained a long-term connection.

Dr. W. felt he was accepting payment for work he was not doing. How could he continue to hold Ms. Pratt's appointments and charge her for the missed ones when he felt he was not really helping her? After exploring the treatment history Dr. W. and I saw that Ms. Pratt indeed had a strong attachment to Dr. W. along with a need to distance him. It was as if she were saying she was afraid to change or to let him know her too well while at the same time she wanted contact based on her needs and on what she could tolerate. Dr. W. questioned whether he was helping Ms. Pratt and whether the twice-a-week sessions were too much. Ms. Pratt did mention every so often that perhaps she should come once a week, but when Dr. W. pursued the question he felt that it would be taken as a rejection if he agreed. He repeated to her at these times that he thought twice-a-week work was important to her. She quickly agreed and for a time she kept appointments regularly.

Sometimes the therapist can't really know what holds a patient in treatment. Years go by and no real change is visible. The therapist despairs or feels guilty that the patient is wasting her money. Is it the therapist's decision to end or cut down the treatment? How does the therapist know for a fact that the money is not well spent? How does the therapist know that if it were not for the treatment the patient would get worse? These were questions we pondered. Dr. W. and I decided that it was in Ms. Pratt's best interest to respect her right to decide about continuing treatment, cutting down, or ending the work.

In *The Analytic Attitude* (1983), Roy Schafer says:

> The adult analysand comes to analysis with a troubled life story, the beginning of which is gradually seen to extend back to earliest child-hood. The formative influences of that early period play a part in vir-tually every important aspect of his or her life. . . . At the core of this formidable problematic life is extreme infantile anxiety or a sense of danger that serves unconsciously as a major rationale for the analysand's ever-present and ever-problematic resistance. Consequently, funda-mental personality change can take place only slowly and in a manner that cannot be predetermined, and an atmosphere of safety can only be developed slowly and uncertainly. [p. 17]

Schafer continues to describe the analytic attitude of empathy, appreciation, and respect that make this work possible. This book is required reading for any technique class I teach.

Considering the patient's pace is always appropriate. In his article "On Beginning Analysis with Borderline Patients"(1990) Michael Porder is firm about telling the "sicker" patient that a com-mitment of four to five times a week is necessary to analytic work. Porder acknowledges that this requirement means that there is significant self-selection among his patients "since those who are too frightened by my recommendation and who wish to be seen less frequently will not continue" (p. 164). What happens to the rest of the patients? As Porder clearly states, the "sicker" patient needs the continuity of frequent sessions. What does the therapist do when faced with a patient who clearly needs four or five ses-sions a week when the patient is willing to be seen only once or twice a week? Porder does not work with a patient who refuses his pre-scription. He says in his excellent paper that only a small percent-age of the patients he sees refuse. It is my feeling that the way Porder tells his patients what they need conveys his conviction and this is what the patients respond to. Those therapists who are not sure about working with a patient, whether consciously or unconsciously, will be less convincing and therefore less likely to be perceived as trustworthy.

The conviction with which the therapist makes a recommendation and then sticks to it is usually tested. It is as if the patient were saying, *"Intimacy frightens me. You couldn't stand to see the real, dirty, murderous me. I'll come here once a week for awhile and then if that seems possible I might try twice. That way we can avoid a close look. We can focus on the outside, on my boss or my boyfriend or even my drug use. My childhood was fine—no need to delve into that. My mother is the only one I've got, for better or for worse. She's part of me and I can't give her up, especially for someone I don't even know. I'd rather evoke feelings in you. I'll bring lots of dreams and be on time and pay on time so you'll like me. Or I'll be so bad about time and money that you'll get distracted and end up not caring if I stay. Or I'll prove that you like me by getting you to call me by my first name or accepting all my phone calls or giving me advice or rearranging my schedule. I'll see that you're afraid of me, and what good are you then? You could never bear my rage and face my pain. After a year or so I'll talk you into letting me cut down or maybe I'll just quit. After all, you failed to show me that I could really trust you."*

As much as the therapist must consider and respect the patient and her pace, she must also and above all trust in the psychoanalytic process. The therapist's ability to convey confidence and conviction and to remain consistent is what the patient needs to feel and see. When the therapist has doubts about working with someone it is helpful to talk with her therapist or a colleague or supervisor. That way the therapist can make her fears conscious, which reduces the chance of acting them out by failing the tests.

A dilemma occurs when the patient is clearly in need of more than one session a week but realistically cannot afford it. Here the therapist must decide whether she is willing and able to reduce the fee or to refer the patient to a clinic, a low-fee referral service, or to a therapist who is able to accept a lower fee. This is an important issue that has an ethical basis. It is really not fair to a patient to deprive her of the treatment of choice and of necessity.

Mrs. Wiley went for a consultation while in treatment with another therapist who worked at a clinic. At the clinic she was seen individually once a week and in a group once a week. Her therapist gave advice and support but this intelligent and disturbed woman realized that something was wrong. She was interested in what was behind her serious depressive episodes. Her therapist at the clinic did not respond to her request to deepen the work. It was clear in the consultation that Mrs. Wiley needed a low fee, and the therapist she consulted with could not accommodate her. Although it is not desirable to refer a depressed patient out, because the rejection can be overwhelming, the therapist had no choice. She told Mrs. Wiley what she thought would be best in a straightforward, tactful manner. The therapist said to Mrs. Wiley that she sounded ready to do the work necessary for a full life and that her intelligence and psychological-mindedness made her a good candidate for psychoanalytic work. The therapist told her this openly and offered to give her the name of someone who was qualified and able to accept a low fee.

As I said above, it is the therapist's conviction that often enables the patient to trust enough to take the therapist's recommendation. The patient also deserves an explanation for the recommended frequency. To paraphrase or quote Porder (1990) cannot do justice to his excellent chapter in *On Beginning an Analysis*, edited by Theodore Jacobs and Arnold Rothstein. Porder's chapter is called "On Beginning Analysis with Borderline Patients" and is required reading for therapists who treat very disturbed patients. Some of the points made in this chapter are:

1. Borderline is not considered to be a specific diagnostic category.
2. After determining that the patient is severely disturbed, propose an "essentially analytic contract" (p. 164) to the patient.
3. Less intensive work puts the patient and therapist at a disadvantage because "therapeutic regression and psychic restructuring is the best treatment for these patients" (p. 164) and frequency allows for continuity of material, which is essential.

4. The beginning of treatment can be intense, chaotic, and confusing.
5. Deal with the massive transference feelings by actively interpreting them, especially when they are projections that are uncomfortable for the patient to own.
6. Suggest to the patient that "much of what he is experiencing with [the therapist] can be understood as aspects of relationships with images of specific people from his past, as aspects of himself which he believes to be in [the therapist], or that he may act toward [the therapist] as he perceived figures from the past had acted toward him" (p. 168).
7. Show the patient, when plausible, that she may be trying to tell the therapist how she felt as a child.

These are only some of the important points Porder makes. His respect for the patient and for the method of intensive psychoanalytic treatment are, in my mind, what make his recommendation for intensive work acceptable to his patients.

Considering and respecting the patient's pace is always necessary and warranted. The psychoanalytically trained therapist learns how to provide her patients with the kind of therapy that can be deepened by listening for the patient's conflicts as they appear, often in disguised ways. Fears about closeness and fears that the therapist is not committed to the process are frequent obstacles in increasing sessions.

CHAPTER 5

Respecting the Patient and the Method

Are patients who have been severely deprived and neglected early in life amenable to psychoanalytic work? Does the consistency of the analytic relationship provide an experience conducive to the development of object and feeling constancy? Can the patient identify with the analyst's function of understanding how the past affects the present? The following cases indicate a resumption of development that occurred as a result of psychoanalytic work. A more supportive therapy with techniques of advice, direction, and guidance may have helped these patients but would not have enhanced their autonomy and therefore their ability to help themselves.

I have consulted with and treated patients who, after years of supportive therapy that included pep talks, advice, and medication, were still at square one in terms of understanding themselves and thereby functioning more independently. It seems to me that giving advice and direction exclusively or even primarily with no attempt to engage a person in understanding her psychodynamics and unconscious fantasy system is disrespectful of the patient's potential for growth.

Miss Webster lived in Philadelphia for many years. She had been depressed for most of her life but managed to earn a living as an actress. At age 21, she sought the help of a psychiatrist who prescribed medication and once-a-week group therapy. The psychiatrist adjusted the medication and gave advice, and the group gave support. Ten years later when Miss Webster's work required that she move to New York she got the name of an analyst from her cousin. The analyst listened to Miss Webster's story and, seeing that she was very disturbed, told her that she would like to see her every day for two weeks, after which time they would decide on a plan. Miss Webster agreed. During those two weeks the analyst assessed Miss Webster's ego functioning, object relatedness, and ability to be self-reflective, along with her symptoms of hypochondriasis and anxiety. She and Miss Webster realized at the end of the two weeks that her previous treatment hadn't touched the deeper issues that were causing her symptoms. The therapist explained to Miss Webster that these symptoms had meaning above and beyond any biological phenomena that might be affecting her, and that she had a right to understand the roots of her difficulties. Miss Webster began analysis and her analyst recently told me that the patient was responding positively. Her hypochondriasis and anxiety had greatly diminished and Miss Webster was using her transference to the analyst to understand herself. Periods of depression were not immobilizing and were connected to the work of mourning losses heretofore unacknowledged. By respecting her patient and the analytic process the analyst was making it possible for Miss Webster to resume development and address certain conflicts that had made her life miserable.

When you respect the patient, everything blossoms. As therapists we learn how to diagnose, how to assess pathology, how to identify defenses, ego deficits, and defects, and how to analyze transference and resistance. We can tend to forget with all of this knowledge that we are meeting a person who has navigated life in ways that deserve our respect as well as our benign curiosity.

With our sophisticated understanding of developmental lines, psychosexual stages, and separation-individuation phases, it becomes clearer and clearer that each person develops uniquely. This information gives a rough schema of normal development but two people with the same experiences (if that were possible) react very differently according to many variables, including constitution. Resilience and the ability to overcome trauma and deprivation are not measurable or predictable. Constitution depends on genetic endowment. The development of the brain depends on so many things—levels of stimulation in early infancy as well as, later on, comfort, nutrition, trauma, both in the pre- and postnatal phases—that IQ in and of itself means relatively little.

Supervising Ms. X. brought this home very clearly. Ms. X. was in supervision as a requirement of her psychoanalytic psychotherapy institute. She worked at an agency for the "intellectually disadvan-taged." I encouraged Ms. X. to select one or two cases to follow and she chose Miss Carter, a 40-year-old mildly retarded woman. Miss Carter had spent her first nine years with her alcoholic mother. She was never sent to school and her home life was reported to be cha-otic, frightening, and filled with deprivation and neglect. Her mother was described as unpredictable and abusive at times but was her only object for many years. It was not known if there were positive times with the mother but, because Miss Carter was articulate and cared for herself in basic ways, we imagined that there were.

When her mother died she went to live with her father and his second wife, a strict, religious woman who used Miss Carter to do her bidding. Mistreatment continued. Miss Carter was physically assaulted, locked out of the house, and told she was ugly and stupid. In school she was tested and put in a class for the retarded. No one considered the effects of trauma and lack of education. When Miss Carter grew up she was sent to a state agency where she applied for and was given the chance to live independently in a supportive apart-ment with roommates and on-site supervision. She did menial work but lost many jobs due to her hyperactivity and combative nature. Counseling was part of the program and luckily Miss Carter's coun-selor was Ms. X.

At first, Miss Carter responded to therapy in her usual infantile manner. She came late or missed appointments, scheduled twice a week at first. She complained incessantly, criticized her therapist, and had tantrums. Ms. X.'s calm, firm, consistent manner combined with empathy and patience had an effect. Luckily for Miss Carter her thera-pist was sophisticated in developmental psychology, open-minded, and aware of the effects of trauma. The agency had only behavior modification in mind for this patient but because Ms. X. was using her case for educational purposes as a requirement of her institute she was given free rein. Ms. X.'s respectful stance and consistent availability, combined with limit setting, was a new experience for Miss Carter. She thrived on it, but there were many tests along the way.

One test took the form of frequent telephone calls. Ms. X. worked with Miss Carter on limiting the phone contact by postulating to Miss

Carter that she was uncertain of Ms. X.'s availability and consistency and used the phone calls to allay her anxiety. She connected Miss Carter's anxiety to her past fears and Miss Carter began to see that her past traumatic life affected the present. Ms. X. asked Miss Carter if she could think of other ways of dealing with her separation anxiety. She avoided giving advice and instead focused on fostering Miss Carter's autonomous functioning. Miss Carter purchased a notebook and sometimes wrote down her feelings. She also took a book to read on the subway and a meditation tape that she found soothing. She began to realize that talking about her feelings eased her panic and after several months she and her therapist agreed to meet four times a week.

The following vignette illustrates Miss Carter's emerging observing ego, ability to differentiate self and object, and beginning empathy for another person.

> *Patient:* My new roommate has a lot of problems. In fact, she has "baby fits" just like I used to have. She reminds me of the way I used to be. Yesterday when I started to yell at her about helping clean the apartment I said to myself, "I have to stop this. I'm treating her just the way my stepmother treated me."

In treating Miss Carter, Ms. X. learned about resilience. She found that given respectful, reliable, and consistent attention Miss Carter gradually began to tell her life story.

As four times a week therapy progressed, Miss Carter began to feel secure enough to start talking about her birth mother. Verbalizing the trauma and attachment was painful but freeing. Before treatment Miss Carter deliberately "forgot" her real mother. As she talked about her early years she began to express anger, feelings of loss and eventually some understanding. Ms. X. refrained from taking sides about Miss Carter's mother, maintaining her neutral stance. This helped Miss Carter retain whatever positive feelings she had about her first object. In the first year of treatment, Miss Carter used splitting to express her feelings.

Patient: [beginning of session] I hate you. I'm so angry at you. Why did you go away? [therapist had canceled an appointment due to illness] I'm not coming here anymore. I don't want to be bothered. You went away and forgot all about me.

Therapist: Your anger takes over and wipes out any other feelings you have.

Patient: [later in session] I don't know how anyone could get angry with you. You're so nice and I have feelings of friendship about you. You're the only person who treats me well. You must be the best therapist there is.

After two years of work, as ambivalent feelings became more tolerable and splitting ebbed, Miss Carter began somatizing as she tried to control her anger. The temper outbursts were replaced by stomachaches and withdrawal during sessions.

Patient: I can't talk today. Friday's session was hard, too.

Therapist: I wonder if you're doing the same thing today, . . . protecting yourself from feeling hurt by not letting yourself feel close to me.

Patient: That's what I did last week. I kept it all inside and then felt sick all weekend. It's because I didn't tell you in words how I felt.

Therapist: I think it gets scary for you to let me know how angry you are when we have a break. You might think your anger would keep me from coming back.

Patient: Must be because I got really angry at my friend for not going to work. I started to yell at her but then I thought about you and your little glasses and red hair and I felt calmer. I went for a walk and felt better.

At the end of the third year Miss Carter was able to work with the transference because the therapist was seen as separate and constant.

Patient: It's like I don't see you on weekends and I think you're far away. I think you might have a house in the country. You go

home after work, pack your bags, and go upstate. I still worry
you might not come back.

Therapist: Is it that fear that I won't come back that makes you
most afraid of our separation?

Patient: Yes. But I think you'd tell me. You're not like my birth
mother—I never knew if or when she would come back. You
won't abandon me.

Here is an illustration of Miss Carter's ability to tolerate and to
use her therapist's abstinent posture.

Patient: I was at a coffee shop yesterday and I thought I saw you.
What color is your coat? [pause] I think you have a red coat. I
wasn't looking for you.

Therapist: What was it like for you to think you saw me outside of
the office?

Patient: I don't know. It was no big deal. But I'm curious, what
would you do if you saw me on the street? I'm just asking a
question. You know all about me. If you saw me would you
come over and talk?

Therapist: I think we can learn more about you if I don't answer
that just yet. What do you think I would do?

Patient: I think you'd ignore me and walk away.

Therapist: So I would act like I didn't know you?

Patient: Yeah. If I saw you and I was with someone, I would say,
"That's a lady I know but we're not related."

Therapist: I think what we're seeing is a growing curiosity about
my life outside of here and a fear that I'd forget about you when
I'm not in the office.

Patient: I guess—a little. Like when you call me back on a weekend I know you're not calling from here. You must be at home.
I wonder what your home is like.

After four years of therapy Miss Carter's therapist left the agency.
There was a long period of preparation for the separation during which
Miss Carter regressed but bounced back and did some remarkable
work.

Patient: I am going to miss you. I can say that. I couldn't before. I have changed and grown up and you have helped me. I am going to miss you.

Therapist: Uh huh.

Patient: I have Ms. B. and Ms. G. to myself but I wish I had two Ms. X.'s. It's just a fantasy. I would keep one of you with me all the time.

Therapist: When you think about me you'll have me with you.

Patient: Yeah. [teary] My fantasy is that you have a very big office at the new place you're going. You have many clients and my fantasy is you'll forget about me.

Therapist: Does that remind you of anything?

Patient: My mother. My mother disappeared and forgot all about me. And my stepmother had babies and never paid attention to me. I used to annoy her to get some attention.

Therapist: So my leaving is bringing back memories of your mother and stepmother.

Patient: Yeah, but if I can think about you, maybe you'll think about me sometimes. I've learned to think about you and try to see you in my mind. Picturing you helps. It calms me down and helps me feel not so lonely.

In summary: Ms. X.'s genuine concern and interest, her benevolent curiosity and the way she was able to make sense out of chaos reached Miss Carter, who all her life had secretly blamed herself for her mother's neglect and abuse. Every abused child holds herself responsible for two reasons. First, the young child sees the world through omnipotent lenses. During this normal developmental phase of omnipotent or magical thinking the child feels responsible for all that happens until a modicum of separation is achieved due to optimal amounts of frustration. Second, as long as the child feels responsible there is hope. It is devastating for a child to realize that what goes on in the world has nothing to do with her. As an adult, however, it is a relief to realize that one is not to blame for a parent's problems. As Miss Carter began to put the pieces of her life together she had her first experience of being an individual with all kinds of feelings.

Over the years Miss Carter's infantile manner of presentation gradually shifted to affective and coherent talk. Our assumption was that she had never been treated with patience and respect in her life. Ms. X.'s ability to be appropriately empathic and noncondescending and to engage the patient in making connections from past to present satisfied the yearning that every human being holds: to be treated decently and with respect and to make sense out of chaos. We also surmised that an identification was taking place with the therapist that began to compete with other less fortunate identifications. A strong bond developed between client and therapist, based at first and exclusively on dependency needs, but which evolved into love and appreciation. Miss Carter was clingy and demanding in the beginning, but as she learned that Ms. X. was reliable and available, object constancy began to develop. She learned to recognize and eventually to consider the needs of others because she allowed herself to feel separate. She learned that she had resources heretofore unused. Ms. X. did not give advice, answer personal questions, or judge Miss Carter's behavior. Instead she tried to engage her in understanding it. We learned that with this new ability to question her reactions, Miss Carter developed frustration tolerance. As she became able to tolerate her own feelings she began to understand that others had feelings too. Her behavior reflected enhanced object relatedness.

Miss Carter never fully caught up in emotional or intellectual development but she grew to the point where she managed to get along with her roommate, to visit her father's family with less emotional upheaval, and to have some pleasure in her life.

Through the process of psychoanalytically oriented psychotherapy Miss Carter came to understand that her past greatly influenced her present. She learned that her initial mistrust of her therapist and others and her fears of closeness and separation were related to her early years. She developed empathy for her difficulty in learning and became more patient with herself and others. She grew to understand that missing first through fifth grades affected her ability to learn. The therapist's listening stance and nondirective approach made it possible for Miss Carter to verbalize and reflect on her feelings. As the process of expressing herself with words became valued, temper tantrums were replaced by the ability to argue. As with all learning there was remarkable growth in self-esteem and self-respect. By identifying and internalizing some of Ms. X.'s qualities Miss Carter blossomed. In terms of structural change, she developed greater ego strengths, enabling her to deal more effectively with her aggression. Her superego became less harsh. Self and object representations softened and new versions competed with more primitive and frustrating ones. Primitive defenses were replaced by more useful and mature ones. It was thrilling to see her develop emotionally and intellectually, development that had been derailed for so long.

The work was deeply moving and taught all concerned—Miss Carter, Ms. X., and me—that being respected and listened to with benevolent curiosity released the potential for growth and development. Putting feelings into words helped Miss Carter resume development and deal with conflicting feelings that had once paralyzed her. She thrived on this treatment—a treatment that would have been denied her, based on her diagnosis. Ms. X.'s respect for her patient and for the psychoanalytic process with its principles of technique were responsible for the important work accomplished.

During the course of our work in supervision Ms. X. also discussed several other patients that she worked with at the agency. The principles of respect, attentive listening, and benevolent curiosity affected all the "intellectually disadvantaged" patients.

For patients who come to therapy with low self-esteem, embarrassment, and shame, being treated in a respectful manner is particularly important. Calling a stranger by her first name can be experienced as infantilizing and even rude.

In a first encounter with a group of ex-heroin users ranging in age from mid-forties to late sixties, in an agency setting, it was natural for me to use Mr., Mrs., or Ms. But, for most of them, it was a new and meaningful experience. These people, some of whom had been in jail, in hospitals, and on welfare, were not used to being treated with respect, and showing them respect helped get the group off to a good start. They shared how important being spoken to as adults was to them. Using psychodynamic principles, the group became a cohesive and ongoing one. The members began to look inside, at the roots of their behavior, and became increasingly able to replace actions with words. Being taken seriously was a first for most of them and they flourished. They became curious about what made them tick and felt rewarded and interested when connections were made between past and present. Talking about their childhood was like dusting off old memories. Whether good or bad, the memories gave these people a new way to see themselves. The past gave the present depth. A new perspective developed.

Mr. Santiago was a thief. He came to the agency because it was a requirement of welfare. Many welfare recipients who were required to come for once-a-week therapy arranged to come for five or ten minutes or skipped appointments once in a while. Not Mr. Santiago. He was prompt and interested in what therapy was about. He kept every appointment when he was not in jail. His therapist was in psychoanalytic training and treated Mr. Santiago using psychoanalytic technique. He listened to his patient's material, pointed out transference phenomena when they were obvious, interpreted resistance when it interfered with treatment, but most of the time he listened. As with Miss Carter and the group of ex-heroin users, Mr. Santiago had never been listened to with benevolent curiosity before.

Over the course of three years Mr. Santiago began to see how his early childhood deprivation and neglect affected him. He began to see that trusting others had never worked out for him, and why he learned to fend for himself as soon as he could. As he began to experience angry feelings and to express them verbally to his therapist he saw that the therapist would not retaliate. This was initially confusing and even frustrating. He could not succeed in provoking his therapist. At first he acted out his frustration and mistrust by getting caught stealing. He served his jail sentence and returned to treatment expecting his therapist to be unavailable. The therapist arranged to resume treatment. Mr. Santiago quite candidly admitted that he let himself be arrested so that he could spend Thanksgiving in jail where he would be served turkey and not feel so alone. Thanksgiving was a holiday for his therapist and, rather than face his feelings about missing his session, Mr. Santiago went to jail. Jail represented a structure, a roof, regular meals, and companionship. Mr. Santiago's therapist asked if this was the whole story. Mr. Santiago associated to the stealing. He began to see that his envy was driving him to take what he could not have. It was easier to steal than to experience the painful envious feelings. The therapist said that Mr. Santiago was in fact feeling his envy by talking about it. The idea of putting feelings into words was a new idea for Mr. Santiago. It fascinated him and he expressed interest in attending group therapy for the first time.

Mr. Santiago's experience in individual therapy opened him to new possibilities. He became more social, more aware of feelings, and more tolerant of others. He developed new skills and interests. He began to feel remorse about taking from others. He found that stealing was less satisfying now that he understood its roots. These changes came about with difficulty. His therapist provided an opportunity by using psychoanalytic technique and by letting Mr. Santiago learn to look inside. Some would say that this improvement was due to a transference cure or a need to please the therapist. Perhaps it was, to some degree, but Mr. Santiago also experienced new ways of relating and improved self-esteem, things that were new to him and that belonged to him for keeps.

Miss O'Hara was not easy to like or to respect. She sought therapy because she wanted to get married. At age 32 she was impatient with waiting for the "right man" to sweep her off her feet. Her good looks, intelligence, sense of humor, and surface charm got her to first base frequently but that was usually the end of the relationship. She had never lived with a man. Dating was as far as she seemed able to go. She went to bed with many men but these were not satisfying experiences, physically or emotionally. She was attracted to men who treated her badly in her eyes. After two or three dates she never heard from them again. When she pursued the relationship she was rebuffed.

Miss O'Hara grew up in the South in an affluent family. She was the youngest of four and her parents were rarely at home. The older siblings teased her and overstimulated her. One brother was sexually provocative but did not abuse her. She loved the attention, but because it was always at such a high pitch she became alternately hyperactive and depressed. Food became her way of self-soothing and she always struggled with weight. At age 13 she discovered amphetamines, which she took regularly.

Dr. A., her therapist, came for consultation because he found himself disliking Miss O'Hara. He could not feel empathic and found himself wanting to advise her rather than understand her. He found her whiny voice and her impatient, entitled attitude particularly annoying. How could he respect her when he found nothing to respect? She was independently wealthy and had never held a job. She dropped out of college and had no interests other than finding a husband. She spent her time shopping.

This is where benevolent curiosity saved the day. Reading Ella Sharpe's (1950) chapters "The Analyst" and "The Analysand," and discussing the case in consultation helped Dr. A. regain his neutral attitude. He relearned that it was not his job to change Miss O'Hara but to try to understand what made her tick and to enlist her curiosity in understanding herself.

He began by saying, as tactfully as possible, that Miss O'Hara's attacking approach was perplexing him. He asked her if she could see what he meant. When she said no he explained. He said, "When you came for therapy you had a rather specific complaint: not being married. Each time you come for a session, instead of exploring and wondering about this, you get angry and impatient with me. I think that you may be behaving with me the same way you behave with other men, and if I'm right we can begin to put the pieces to this puzzle together."

Miss O'Hara reacted with some interest and caution.

Patient: You mean that *I* have something to do with the problem?

Therapist: Well, if you think about it, it is a possibility.

Patient: But I pay *you* to solve the problem. What am *I* supposed to do?

Therapist: You can start by thinking of our work as a collaboration. As you tell me about your thoughts and feelings—your dreams when you remember them—we'll start to learn some of the things that frighten you or worry you. The best way to do that is to relax and say what comes to mind.

Patient: That sounds foolish to me but I guess I can try it. When I left home today I forgot my checkbook so I can't pay you. I know I was supposed to pay last time but I promise to bring my checkbook Friday. Is that okay?

Therapist: It's okay but I think it might be helpful to see what comes to mind about forgetting your checkbook.

Patient: Nothing comes to mind. I just forgot.

Therapist: See if you can let your thoughts wander and say what occurs to you.

Patient: Last time I was here you told me you would be away next week. You didn't tell me why and I thought you were rude.

Therapist: Sounds like you were annoyed and perhaps that's why you don't feel like paying me today.

Patient: Well, it's possible, but I don't really expect you to be any different than other men. None of them can be counted on. Even my brothers let me down.

Therapist: How?

Patient: They left home, that's how! Especially Tim—he was the closest to me and he knew how lonely I'd be but he went off to college and left me in that empty house with no one but the servants.

Therapist: Tell me about it.

Miss O'Hara began talking about what it was like at home and, possibly for the first time in her life, she was listened to quietly and attentively. She remarked at the end of the session on how quickly the time had passed.

I've tried to illustrate with this vignette that sometimes it is difficult for the therapist to feel any rapport with the patient. The patient picks up the therapist's frustration or dislike, and the two parties find themselves feeling hostile towards each other. Whether this is purely transference and countertransference, testing, or a bad match is not always easy to say. If the therapist remembers that the job is to understand, and not to solve problems or cure them, a lot of pressure is alleviated. Benevolent curiosity is enormously helpful in situations where patient and therapist clash or can't communicate.

This is not to say that a therapist can work with every patient. We all have our limitations, and sometimes making a referral to someone else is necessary. Such a decision involves respecting the patient enough to see that she gets the best possible treatment. Making such a referral will be taken as a rejection by the patient but if done tactfully and sincerely, with as much explanation as we are capable of giving, it is in the patient's best interest.

Dr. L. came to supervision with a case he was ready to give up on. His patient, Mr. Freed, had been in analysis for two years and nothing was happening. Mr. Freed repeatedly came late, even after rearranging appointments to suit him. Dr. L. was wondering if indeed his patient was analyzable. He acknowledged that he was losing interest in the case. I looked at this reaction as induced countertransference. The patient was succeeding in pushing his analyst away to defend against looking beneath his somewhat happy-go-lucky façade. After talking about his patient, Dr. L. and I saw that this man was extremely anxious about his secret fantasy life. Mr. Freed had never married. His relationships with women were short-lived and unsatisfying. His free time was spent going to the Off Track Betting parlor and, when he could afford it, he went to Atlantic City to gamble. Dr. L. and I conjectured that the patient had a perverse structure that gave him enough pleasure to avoid or suppress his pain.

Because of Mr. Freed's history of addictive behavior and his difficulty in getting to sessions, Dr. L. questioned his initial recommendation of analysis. What does the analyst do when in this kind of doubt? Dr. L. and I felt that Mr. Freed had to be engaged in the decision of whether to continue analysis or to shift to a less intensive mode of work. In my opinion, this is a most difficult dilemma. Telling a patient that analysis is not the treatment of choice after recommending it is authoritarian and sounds punitive. My hope would be to work on deepening the treatment gradually, using the visible transference manifestations.

When treatment comes to a standstill as in this case, I listen for the transference message. The loudest and clearest message was acted out by lateness, and enacted by both parties in the dyad seeming to lose interest in and hope for the analysis. Due to certain dreams and material I wondered if homosexual fantasies were being denied or avoided. This is not at all unusual in psychoanalytic work because everyone has homosexual and heterosexual fantasies that are frequently unconscious. How to bring them to consciousness and how to give the patient some insight into the difficulty requires skill, tact, and timing. With Mr. Freed I might have said something like, "I wonder if your lateness, which you seem to be unable to make sense of or to conquer, has to do with a discomfort in spending more time with me." Exploring why this situation existed by looking at what was happening in treatment would shed light on things. I would say something like, "Often, embarrassment about sexual thoughts and feelings between people whether between men, or men and women, or women and women cause people to distance themselves rather than acknowledge them." Such an intellectual interpretation is usually not wise but when treatment reaches an impasse and when enough material is available it can be relieving to a patient. It lets the patient know that the therapist is not shocked and can deal with sexual material in a nonjudgmental, comfortable way. There were enough references in the process recordings to indicate anxiety about man-to-man closeness. This material, along with the patient's distant and disappointing relationship with a cold father, its repetition in the transference, and the possibility of a stalemate, made such an interpretation plausible.

What does all this have to do with respecting the patient? I have been in classes and seminars, and read articles where patients with perverse structures have been deemed unanalyzable. Theoretically, the perverse activity provides gratification that is ego-syntonic, and not enough "neurotic" suffering occurs. Also, perversion is seen as a preoedipal solution. Many analysts, particularly those trained thirty or more years ago, see analysis as a treatment for oedipal conflicts only. This seems more along the lines of a value judgment. People are too complex to make such assessments quickly. The pioneering work of Leo Stone (1954), Hans Loewald (1960), and Phyllis Green-acre (1970) has changed the idea that analysis is only for the so-called neurotic patient.

The stance of respectful, benevolent curiosity saves us from jumping to conclusions about who is suitable for analytic work. It is the patient who must decide if a second chance is worth looking inside at issues that are often painful and frightening. It is the therapist's job to help the patient understand and analyze the obstacles or resistance, and to provide a safe environment, to respect the patient's right to look deeper, and to provide a method to do so.

❖ C H A P T E R   6 ❖

Separations between Patient and Therapist

Separations between patient and therapist are crucial times in terms of deepening psychoanalytic work. Such times evoke memories of past separations in the patient's life—times that always have a valence of pain. Feelings of abandonment, loneliness, rage, anxiety, sadness, and powerlessness that we all felt in infancy and childhood resurface. When these feelings can be articulated a shift occurs, but when the feelings bypass conscious awareness they are acted out and can threaten the therapy itself. This is why the therapist must listen and watch for signs of the patient's pain and anxiety. Pre-vacation time and post-vacation time are opportunities to deepen the treatment and for growth to occur.

Every patient I have worked with and every case I have supervised or consulted on has impressed me with how deeply separations are felt. If not dealt with and interpreted, reactions to separations (often unconscious at first) can herald the end of therapy.

Separations include weekends, one missed or canceled appointment, or a six-week vacation. Feelings are evoked no matter who is responsible for the separation—patient or therapist. For therapists who take time off in August, the Memorial Day weekend is the time to start listening for separation themes and references. July 4th is another holiday that sets off feelings about the August break.

Because troubled patients often need to deny the separateness of the therapist, the therapist's vacation is particularly distressing. The patient is faced with the irrefutable fact that she does not and cannot control the therapist and that the therapist has a separate life.

Before presenting case material here are some practical matters to think about:

Announcing a Planned Absence It is important to give the patient as much notice as possible. I announce my summer vacation plans when I begin working with a patient. This is because I have always taken time in August. If the therapist is not sure, three months notice seems workable. This gives patients time to co-ordinate their vacations with their therapists. If a patient has just begun treatment and has already made plans that do not coincide with mine I respect this and do not charge.

Leaving a Message On Your Answering Machine Most therapists say something like, "This is Dr. X. I will be away from the office until September 2. I will be getting my messages several times a week and will call you back as soon as possible. In case of emergency please call Dr. Y. at ————." or "This is Mrs. A. I will be back in the office on September 2. Please call back then, or if you wish to speak to a therapist immediately please call Mr. Q." I give the name of a covering therapist to those patients who want or may need one before I leave.

Unplanned Absences When the absence is brief, common sense is the best guide. It is important to refrain from giving reasons to most patients who are doing analytic work because burdening a patient with facts can preclude an important chance for fantasy (see Chapter 1).

What to Tell the Patient During the consultation phase I tell patients that I take several vacations a year, a month during the summer and two weeks in spring or winter. I say that I will give ample advance notice and ask that they coordinate their vacations with mine.

Consistency If at all possible it is best to take the summer break at the same time each year. This provides the important rhythm and consistency so helpful in psychoanalytic work.

Personal Emergencies Long illnesses and other emergencies must be thought through and acted on according to the situation. If the analyst must be away from the office for no more than a month or two, most patients who are doing analytic work will wait. If the patient is just beginning treatment or is very fragile, the therapist can offer a referral or someone to see in the meantime. Because respecting the patient's autonomy is so important it is wise to engage the patient in such a decision when possible. If the patient must cancel sessions for a long stretch of time the therapist need not hold the hours open but can offer what available hours she has after the break in treatment. This way it is not necessary to charge for the missed appointments.

The Last Session before a Long Break When a patient introduces new material in the last session I make a bridging comment like, "This is certainly something for us to take up in the fall." It is hard to do justice to a new theme in one session and common sense tells us to wait. I always shake hands before a long break and again when treatment resumes. This probably has to do with custom and tradition but I have found that patients seem to welcome this personal contact. I did when I was in treatment.

I will present case material with the aim of illustrating work done prior to the August vacation. The thoughts and interventions are based on years of work between patient and therapist. Readers will hear the following material from different angles and will think of the multiple meanings in the vignettes. There is a shared pool of data when two people spend time together on an ongoing basis over a long period of time. The therapist brings her own associations to the work and a series of bridges are created that are meaningful to the two parties. Whenever reading case material the reader brings her own associations based on her past and her unconscious. This process is personal and it is why therapists with similar training hear and respond to the same case material differently. Case seminars and group supervision are valuable for the therapist for new light is shed on cases, and blind spots for one therapist are spotted by another therapist. Ongoing supervision is valuable in deepening understanding by spotting countertransference and by observing parallel process. My experience supervising and being supervised has led me to respect the ways different people relate to the material. No two therapists hear or think alike, but all roads do lead to Rome. The journeys differ depending on the travelers, but it is the journeys that count.

The first patient had been in treatment for five years at the time of the following excerpts of sessions. The patient, Ms. Stevens, is a 33-year-old lawyer, recently divorced. The first session is on July 5th, right after a long holiday weekend.

SESSION 1

Patient: I had a dream the opposite of my "late" dreams. I was ready and everyone else was late. I was at a business meeting and I had important information to share but I couldn't get everyone together. I cleared off the table but no one came. I was waiting. I had such important stuff to tell them and no one listened. I barely recognized myself. I was a thin, small, dark person [the analyst has dark hair] with glasses. Very bookish and businesslike—no sense of humor, intense and nasty [patient is blond, often bubbly with a good sense of humor]. I was like a composite of my sister and mother and a friend. I was small and bossy.

Associations: Yesterday I was off. Bob [boyfriend] was away and Lois came over to watch fireworks from the roof. In the dream I was completely frustrated and intent on getting my own way. Bob was late. I waited for him. No one cared. People were ignoring me and focused on other things. It felt like me but it wasn't me. Nothing else occurs to me. [pause] Not a very interesting dream. The feeling was me alone against everyone else. At work I feel alone, and even watching fireworks with Lois I was alone because everyone else was at the barbecue. I'm jealous of my ex-husband's new house. How dare he!

Therapist: You're angry at feeling alone and left—with no one paying attention.

Patient: I want more attention from Bob, so I'm nice and pleasant when we're together. At work I suppress my huffiness and lately I've been getting attention.

Therapist: What are your feelings about here and me? I'll be going away soon.

Patient: I don't feel bad. No one can fix my alone feeling, not even Bob. I can't subject anyone to it.

Therapist: It sounds like you're saying that you can't subject me to your feelings. But that's why you're here and your dream expresses feelings.

Patient: You can't do anything to fix it. That's why I used to use pot. Smoking took it away for a while. I have to bear it 'til it goes away. In the dream my behavior was turning people off. I have to bear it.

In this session Ms. Stevens reiterates her feeling that she must be nice so people (the analyst) will not turn away. The theme of being left and kept waiting is stated and the therapist reminds the patient that she will be away on vacation soon. The patient expresses doubt about sharing her anger directly and is more comfortable blaming her ex-husband.

SESSION 2

Patient: I had a dream with another new theme: people trying to hurt me physically. The dream felt so real that I was glad to wake up. Strangers were attacking me. They know why but I don't. A dark-haired woman was putting green gum on my teeth. I made her take it off. I was in an apartment where people did bad things to people. There were dead bodies in the closet. I talked my way out. I managed to fend them off. They were cannibals or torturers. Not the way I am. They had the capacity to keep me but I won out. This is the way I am with men and everyone. I want to be told what to do and I want to tell them what to do. I want to be powerful and to be overpowered. With Bob I'll do anything if he pleases me. Oral sex, anal sex, anything. I wait on him. It's scary because after a while it would be like he's the pimp and I'm a prostitute. I would be his slave and I could keep him—hold on to him—hold on to his affection and attention. It's a means to an end. If I could be

100 percent sure of no disease I would screw anyone and every-one—for money, I could do what I like and be paid for it. It would be pure pleasure and profit. I would be in control and no one could leave me. It reminds me somehow of the movie, *The Picture of Dorian Gray.* An evil, violent part of me that I must hide. It's my job to keep it hidden so I won't hurt some-one. It's the only way to protect the ones I love.

Therapist: You protect me by keeping an emotional distance. You're afraid to show me your anger about my being in con-trol about my vacation.

Patient: Something's going on. It's hard to talk about. It feels like *TheTwilight Zone* when a man saw a monster on the wing of the plane and no one else could see it. The man was trying to warn the pilot. I have a horrible monster and I can't control it when I sleep. When I used to be depressed I don't remember this fear. I was just unhappy and withdrawn. This other side of me is not benign. I'm afraid of losing my temper—being out of control.

Therapist: You can express these feelings with words, and if you lose control I will tell you that you can take a deep breath and we'll understand what set you off.

Patient: I want you to reach in and cure it. It's the ugliest thing I've ever seen just because of the way it makes me feel. I'm loath to lean on you. And even if I can't do anything bad in here I'm afraid of unleashing it when I'm alone and when you're away.

In this session Ms. Stevens recognized that the people trying to hurt her represented an aspect of herself. She began to acknowledge how upset she was about being left and to what lengths she'd go to stay in control. Later in treatment Ms. Stevens referred to this session as "meeting the monster" in herself. The session reflects the patient's need to sexualize her wishes for closeness. The cannibal references let the patient and therapist see that the rage had roots in the oral phase of development. This information was used later on and had the effect of helping the patient understand the strength and roots of her feelings, thereby lessening her fear and embarrassment in the present. The therapist says that it is safe to express her feelings, indicating that she is not afraid of anything the patient might say. The patient's wish to have the therapist reach in and fix the ugliness means several things. To touch an ugly monster means not being afraid or repulsed and can be seen as a caring gesture. The patient is also using a passive mode to shift her fantasized omnipotence to the therapist.

SESSION 3

Patient: I hate you and I hate this process. I want to be here but I don't want to talk. I know about your vacation and I don't want to discuss it. I think I've reached the extent of what I can do here and I want to stop. You never agree.

Therapist: You're exploring new feelings and you're angry that I'm leaving next week.

Patient: That may be true but I can't continue. After all these years of this hard work you still leave me—and with all of these new feelings. How can you! How can you keep calling the shots— saying when and for how long? Even though I'll save time and money when you're away, what happens if something goes wrong? I only have my friends. [angry pause] How much will it take for you to give up on me?

Therapist: You fear your anger will put me off or frighten me. Talking about your anger is important.

Patient: I'm frustrated with myself. Two months before you leave whatever is inside of me surfaces and then I have to shut down. Bob is going away for a week, too. I wonder how I got into this. I hate feeling attached to you. I had a fantasy that I could give you a postcard, self-addressed and stamped, and you could mail it. Lois does that with her son at camp.

Therapist: You're saying that you'll miss me and when you miss people it keeps them closer than if you forget them.

Patient: How can I know if you miss me? You go away every year at this time. This time seems the worst.

Therapist: I guess in some ways it feels worse, but letting yourself feel close to someone is different from feeling alone.

In this session Ms. Stevens expresses her anger and despair directly to the therapist. At first she wants to end treatment—to leave the therapist instead of being left. She says that after all these years of complying with the therapist and giving new material she still can't control her. The therapist talks about how missing someone, though painful, can keep the missed person close by thinking about them. (This is a technique reinforcing object constancy—thinking about the lost object keeps her close. I am always reminded of the very sad moment at the end of the movie *E.T.* when Elliott is saying goodbye. E.T. touches Elliott's head with his finger and says, "I'll be right here.")

SESSION 4

Patient: I'm feeling much friendlier to you and even relaxed about your vacation. Last year I wouldn't picture you with anyone at all. This year I've given you a friend and a dog in my fantasy. Something must have happened. Why do I feel so much better about you? I remember last year it was hot in here and I asked you to turn on the air conditioner in an angry way. You said it was broken. Today it's not on and I don't feel that wave of hostility. I don't feel choked up with impatience. It's mysterious the way I feel better. I don't want to be that difficult child anymore. All I needed was a lot of patience. Things could have turned out so differently if my mother had been patient. I guess it's useless to ask you what made the difference.
Therapist: What do you remember about last time?
Patient: I got the feeling that you would think of me once in a while on your vacation. And I know I can think of you whenever I want.

These sessions illustrate the value in expressing anger in words. Dreams and fantasies of sadistic anger were verbalized and partially understood. The therapist remained calm and patient. By asking Ms.

Stevens what she remembered about the last session the therapist introduced the idea of remembering—of *feeling constancy*. This was by no means the end of Ms. Stevens's anger, but her ability to calm herself with the idea that thoughts about a person keep her near helped her tolerate the summer break. Ms. Stevens saw that her anger could not kill or even frighten the therapist.

If the patient can express anger before the vacation, resuming work after the break is easier. Sometimes patients find it too difficult to express the anger of abandonment or loss before the break and must wait until the therapist returns safely. I have also noticed that some patients become anxious about the therapist's welfare before a break. I have said to some patients, "Don't worry, I'll be fine." This is meant to tell the patient that her anger will not destroy me.

> Ms. Simon came to a therapist in a depressed state. Her husband had left her and she was distraught, blaming herself for pushing him away. After working twice a week for a year the therapist, Dr. L., had to cancel two weeks of sessions without much notice. When he returned Ms. Simon announced that she had made a big decision. She had decided to apply to graduate school out of state. Dr. L. noticed his patient's improved mood and felt the decision was a healthy one (value judgment replaced benign curiosity). Ms. Simon informed him that she had to cut down to once a week in order to save money. Dr. L. asked if she was sure about her decision and when she said yes he agreed to see her once a week until she left for school in six months. Several weeks later Ms. Simon left treatment without notice. What happened? Dr. L. failed to help Ms. Simon explore her reactions to his sudden cancellations. This is a major error because an important opportunity was passed up. Separations between patient and therapist always evoke feelings. If treatment is to deepen, these feelings must be acknowledged and worked with.

Had the therapist in Ms. Simon's case asked her to talk about her decision to cut down before he agreed, and had he listened for her anger about the recent break in treatment, Ms. Simon might have been able to see that her anger or sense of loss had something to do with her decision. Even if the connection remained obscure to Ms.

Simon she would have heard her therapist's words as indicating that he was not afraid of her anger and was curious about the timing of her decision. His quick willingness to agree with her wish to cut down implied that he did not care. Had there been no separation Ms. Simon's sudden decision might have been viewed by the therapist as resistance. But a patient's sudden decision to stop treatment often has to do with a perceived or real action of the therapist's with the decision to cut down or quit as retaliation. In reviewing the case Dr. L. remembered that Ms. Simon had made him sleepy during many sessions. Upon further exploration he realized that his sleepiness was an unconscious response to fears about her hostility and possible psychotic rage. This is an example of unconscious communication between patient and therapist. The patient decides to reduce her sessions and eventually quits therapy (action takes the place of thought.) The therapist agrees (decision based on an unconscious fear of the patient, which made him sleepy). Abrupt endings in therapy are often the result of such enactments (unconscious repetitions and communications) between patient and therapist. It is noteworthy that Ms. Simon's presenting problem centered on her fear that she had pushed away her husband.

When a change in schedule is announced either by patient or therapist, there are bound to be feelings. Even when a patient asks the therapist to change an appointment and the therapist agrees there is often a negative reaction that must be explored. After rescheduling a patient at his request because of a business meeting, the patient, Mr. Young, expressed annoyance. We learned that my doing him a favor made him feel uncomfortable for he felt that he would be indebted to me. It made him angry that I had the power to grant his request.

Separations always affect the patient although this is most often denied. We are used to hearing a patient say, "I can hardly wait until your vacation. I'll save money and have time to myself," or "I forgot when you said you were leaving; it can't be soon enough for me," or "I've decided to take my vacation the week after you return (or the week before you leave)."

The therapist cannot overlook such statements or take them at face value. But what can the therapist say in the face of such adamant denial that her presence is in any way important? I say something like, "There's no doubt that you're pleased about not paying and having more time but I wonder if there are other feelings too" (benevolent curiosity).

Mrs. Flynn claimed to have no other feelings about the therapist's vacation but several weeks before the break she began reporting thoughts of ending treatment and having an extramarital affair. The therapist asked her to look at why she wanted to leave right before the vacation break. She realized that it would be easier to leave than to be left. The affair was meant to replace the therapist rather than face the feelings of missing him. These realizations did not come quickly. Sessions were spent on feelings about separations, past and present. Mrs. Flynn accused the therapist of making a mountain out of a molehill. Because of his experience he persisted in connecting her lateness and thoughts of ending therapy to the vacation. The therapist knew that Mrs. Flynn had intense reactions to arbitrary authority, and although she had put her therapist on a pedestal his days there were numbered. When Mrs. Flynn paid her July bill she forgot to sign his check. This slip helped her see that there were indeed mixed feelings about the vacation.

If a patient forgets to pay the bill, or comes late after a separation is announced, these actions can be seen as equivalents of anger and anxiety. It is not at all unusual for patients to skip sessions or threaten to end treatment after the therapist has returned from vacation. In such instances the treatment can be deepened if new light is shed on the feelings about the interruption of treatment.

Here are excerpts from sessions following a four-week vacation break from Mrs. Birch, a patient who had decided before the vacation to increase her sessions from three to four times a week after the summer break.

SESSION 1

Patient: [smiling, shakes hands] Am I glad to see you! [lies on the couch] I had an awful time—thought of you constantly. I picked fights with everyone. My mind is going in a million directions.

At one point I thought I was having a nervous breakdown so I taught Susie [daughter] to play backgammon. I wanted to call you a lot. I promised myself I would tell you . . . I'm going to cut down. I have so many expenses—I need so many things. I realize analysis won't end soon and I can't keep depriving myself in the meantime. I need to see the dentist, the gynecologist, I need clothes. All essential things. I needed you and you weren't there. That's fucked up. There was not another person or thing that could take your place. This is shattering and scary. I hated your guts. You could have told me where you were. You didn't have to go. You should indulge me. Now I want to hold you at arm's length. It's my need and my option. I don't want to suffer like that again. If getting close causes such pain I don't need it. It's like whipping headlong into a tunnel I don't know about. I feel young, childish, naïve. [crying]

The therapist told the patient that she had relived something from her past during the break. This intrigued her but she remained firm about her decision to cut down. The therapist interpreted her fear of closeness and how she defended against it with reality pressures. He told the patient that this was her analysis and that it would make her treatment very difficult for her if she cut back instead of increasing sessions as they had agreed to do.

SESSION 2

Patient: I looked at the cartoons in the waiting room. I'm excited today because of yesterday's session and also that you're back. By the way, when you were gone I had fantasies of having affairs with other men. It was a need thing. I wanted to get involved with Charlie. Not in reality. I wanted to pull in and keep away. It was a replacement for you in a way. I wanted to play with him—fool around. I have a need for him to want me . . . to need me . . . to engulf me . . . to be there every day.

Therapist: I see Charlie as representing me, but you're having difficulty feeling your wishes for closeness here, with me.

Patient: Is it really such a terrible thing to cut down? I'm afraid you'd withdraw.

Therapist: You seem to be afraid that if you need me I will withdraw so you talk about withdrawing first. [He goes on to say that in her decision to cut down was a wish that he would feel the way she felt when he announced his vacation.]

Patient: You're making it very hard for me. I really want to see you every day.

SESSION 3

Patient: All right! I won't cut down [sarcastic]. How nice that you're right and I'm wrong. You're safe and I run around like a raw nerve. I feel embarrassed and humiliated. Sure it's my analysis but it's like cutting off an arm to save the rest of the body. [crying] I'm glad I'm becoming aware and can feel the pain instead of taking drugs or smoking pot like I used to do. [She continues to berate the therapist.] What do I have to do to make you feel the pain? I want to hurt you. How much pain do I have to go through? You can't know how much it took for me to reach this decision. So now what! Why can't you give me something?

Therapist: If you could feel right now that I did understand how difficult this is, it would mean feeling closer and this is exactly what you're fighting.

Here the therapist could have stayed with the anger but he chose to interpret what lay beneath it.

SESSION 4

Patient: [two minutes late] Well, this is the infamous fourth hour. I was talking to Nina and the time went by so fast. I didn't tell

Bob [husband] at first. I told him I was working late. When I did tell him he was angry. How can I feel close to you with demands? You have it all your way. You're so strong.

She went on to associate to being told she was a big girl when her baby brother was born and she knew she wasn't. Other memories of unfair treatment and rejection came up along with the idea that girls in her family came second to the boys. She began to acknowledge envy of her brothers. "Just because they had penises they were treated better."

In presenting these clinical vignettes I have tried to illustrate that separations between patient and therapist are always to be taken seriously. It is not at all uncommon for patients to want to cut down or stop treatment after a vacation. The therapist's job is to interpret this wish as a reaction to feelings about the separation, which are traceable to past feelings of abandonment or rejection. The wish to cut down or quit can also be seen as a test on the patient's part to determine if the therapist can tolerate intense neediness.

Separations mean different things to different patients at different times during therapy. First of all, knowing that the therapist has something else to do can be upsetting. Some patients like to picture the therapist as never leaving her chair or office. When she does, it means she has another life. The roots of the wish for the ever-present therapist are obvious. No child enjoys sharing a parent or loved one. This idea of sharing usually brings to mind the idea of the therapist's spouse, or child, or significant other, although Miss Stevens would only picture her therapist with a dog and a friend. It took several years of treatment for her to give the therapist a family in her fantasy.

The following material is from two different patients and is meant to illustrate how ambivalence is expressed through oral wishes to devour. The vignettes occur during the week before the analyst's August vacation and show that the wish to devour serves to hold onto the analyst lovingly and to destroy the analyst hatefully.

The first patient is a 30-year-old woman in an analysis that began as psychotherapy.

Patient: I had a dream: I was at an inn with my boyfriend, and the bread that was served was cooked or baked with dead people's parts. I don't want to confront this. It's childish, primitive. [B, the patient, and E, the boyfriend, are both facing the August break in analysis.] I told the dream to E even though I should have told you first. I realize I dilute it that way. I found the dream eerie. It had a big effect on me. I felt scared when I realized the bread was made of dead people. I saw the innkeepers as evil people. It had the elements of a fairytale—Hansel and Gretel come to mind. Their parents left them in the woods.

Therapist: You have parents leaving their children.

Patient: Yeah! That must have to do with you analysts leaving us. But it's so childlike, this dream.

Therapist: You have feelings about me leaving.

Patient: When I was a kid I saw a play about a huge ogre who ate his children. It's like the innkeepers and the parents are absolute evil. I like everything to be black and white. I want explanations for everything.

Therapist: Like how can I go away and leave you?

Patient: Your leaving reminds me of kindergarten, when my mother left me at school or at camp. I'm afraid now like I was then about the unknown.

Therapist: So if you eat someone up they can't leave you . . . they're still with you.

Patient: Yes, maybe that's what the dream is about—or if I can't have you no one else can. But I didn't do the killing in the dream.

Therapist: It was your dream and it expresses your feelings through the different characters.

The second patient is a 50-year-old accountant in her tenth year of analysis, who has arranged to have plastic surgery during the August break.

Patient: I had the worst nightmare. I woke up and looked to see if there was a killer—a man with a knife.

Therapist: You've been talking about the surgery you're having when I'm away.

Patient: Yes, I wanted to know if the anesthesia would be general. I've heard that can be dangerous.

Therapist: Dangerous.

Patient: People die from that.

Therapist: You're frightened and you've replaced me with another doctor.

Patient: In the dream I killed someone—a woman [therapist is a woman]. I went to a restaurant where the customers ordered by pointing to the food that was in the shape of flayed women. Breasts, waists, and thighs like frogs' legs. Even the fruit was shaped like that. They were killing women customers for dinner—you could see their husbands and boyfriends panicking. The dream was on Saturday and the next night I wanted to go to Sue and John's so I wouldn't have to be alone. [In a previous session the patient spoke of Sue and John, who were getting married, and how jealous she felt.] They're moving next week and I'm jealous about that. Reminds me of my parents.

Therapist: I'll be "moving" next week to go on vacation. I think it's connected.

Patient: I have no control over anyone. People always go off and leave me and they have each other and I'm alone. And with you—it's like you're dead when you leave. I can't call you or even know where you are. I have no say in it. On the way here I was angry with you.

Therapist: And anger can make you want to kill. You make me dead rather than think of where I'll be or who I'm with. That deprives you of me so in the dream you eat me up.

Patient: That sounds gross. Disgusting. I feel sick.

Therapist: Everyone's earliest experiences center on eating. A baby sees the world through its mouth. It takes in what it wants and spits out what it doesn't want.

Patient: I feel like Orwell's *1984*—completely out of control. Everyone is bigger and stronger and doing their thing. [crying] I wonder if I had these thoughts about my mother. Did I want to eat her up or spit her out?

Therapist: Probably both. Babies have mixed feelings and so do adults. You want me to stay with you and your angry self wants me dead. Perhaps there's a compromise.

Patient: I suppose I could think about you having a nice rest. Not fun, just rest. At least that way you'll come back to me.

Powerful and primitive feelings are evoked by impending separation. Both patients were able to work with their cannibalistic urges and the oedipal jealousy expressed in their dreams. They were able to see that their present anger had roots in the past. Working through intense feelings in the transference repeatedly is a chance afforded by the uniqueness of analysis. The intensity of therapy permits a reliving of the past in the present with the analyst as transference object and as a new, nonretaliating, patient person who can help make connections from past to present.

When treating more troubled patients the therapist is often faced with the dilemma of how to respond to a patient's decision to postpone or end treatment. A colleague contributed the following vignette.

While on vacation the analyst received a message on his tape that Miss Martinelli would not be resuming treatment in September as planned but due to her rehearsal schedule (she was an actress) she would begin in October. Because she had left treatment two weeks before the therapist's August vacation it meant that the break entailed a separation of nine weeks. Miss Martinelli's message did not invite the analyst to call her back. The therapist was sure, based on their prior work, that she was acting out her anger and her need to be in charge. He also saw the action as a test. Miss Martinelli's parents had been self-involved people who, by never setting limits for their five children, deprived them of feeling cared for. The analyst felt that by not responding to Miss Martinelli's message he would be repeating the parental attitude of not caring. Nine weeks is a long break in analytic work and Miss Martinelli's object constancy was problematic. The analyst felt that whatever he did would be a mistake. If he called her he would not be respecting her autonomy; if he did not call he would be experienced as not caring. How could he pass this test?

The analyst decided to wait until he was back from vacation and then called Miss Martinelli. Because she was in analysis he felt his role was to interpret; however, without the patient nothing can happen. In this case the patient did not respond to the phone message and in fact left treatment by not returning. The analyst wrote a note saying that he felt talking about things would be important. The note left the door open and also let the patient know she had not killed him off. Six months later Miss Martinelli made an appointment. She told the analyst that the note meant a lot to her but her schedule had been too hectic to respond. After several sessions she acknowledged how hurt and angry she was at him for leaving and she eventually connected these feelings to her father's death. A period of mourning followed, mourning that had been avoided for many years.

Sometimes patients don't return after a separation. The therapist can only hope that the work done prior to the interruption of treatment will remain in some corner of the patient's mind. Unfinished business often makes a more indelible impression than completed work.

Tolerating the Patient's Rage

The therapist's ability to tolerate the patient's expression of rage is one of the most difficult and important tests she must pass when doing psychoanalytic work. I have learned through my own experience and from supervising others that the patient's expression of anger towards the therapist is often unconsciously discouraged by the therapist.

Because it is not easy to be the recipient of intense anger the therapist must remind herself that accepting and understanding it is a top priority. Tendencies to be helpful, caring, and empathic are required of the psychotherapist, but when these tendencies are used to avoid the patient's rage they can inhibit the development of the transference and the deepening of treatment. Learning how to remain empathic while at the same time remaining firm is an ongoing process for the therapist. Real empathy includes being firm and consistent enough for the patient to express anger. What is unique about the analytic situation is that the patient's expression of anger is never responded to in kind. Because the anger has never been tolerated before, it often takes years of testing for the patient to understand that it is safe to express it. Many of these patients had parents or caretakers who ignored them or retaliated harshly when frustration was expressed. As children such patients learned to be "good" and noncomplaining. Some found outlets for the anger in delinquency, sadistic behavior to other children or animals, accident-proneness, and drug abuse. Masochistic character styles and symptoms are indicators of buried rage. Such patients often succeed in getting others, including the therapist, to feel and behave sadistically towards them.

It is the nonverbalized, acted-out anger that often ends the treatment. This acted-out anger is far more destructive to the treatment than the verbalized anger. It affects the therapist in a very different way. When a patient behaves self-destructively, for instance, the therapist is made to feel helpless, worried, responsible, and often angry. It is at times like these that much skill and tact is required. The therapist must alert the patient to the anger and to the fact that the patient is so uncomfortable with it that she would rather the therapist feel and express it. At such times I have said something like, "I wonder if you're aware that right now you're trying to get me to feel angry so that you can avoid feeling it?" or "It seems that it feels safer to you if I feel angry instead of you feeling angry." Such explanations must be made repeatedly over time with calmness and patience so that the sadomasochistic enactment can be analyzed. It is not at all unusual for the masochistic patient to enrage the therapist. When the therapist begins losing patience she must find ways to interpret the enactment to the patient.

When a patient is behaving in a self-destructive way she is often saying to the therapist, "You are powerless to help me. You are ineffective. You are failing me. You are worthless." This message is most often indicative of the patient's feelings of helplessness and failure. The therapist must interpret this message, for if it is not deciphered the chance of a stalemate is great. This is an aspect of what some call a *negative therapeutic reaction*, where the treatment goes on and on and the patient gets worse or makes no gains.

In the fifth year of treatment Joe (mentioned in Chapter 1) began abusing Valium after a long period of not using drugs. I tried to analyze the action to no avail. One day I told him that I would not continue his analysis unless he stopped harming himself and joined me in understanding what he was feeling. He sat up on the couch and sobbed. My ultimatum, he said, proved that I cared about him more than my fee. He checked into a hospital for help in withdrawing and resumed the analytic work after several months. The Valium use was explored and turned out to be multidetermined. One aspect was Joe's fear of experiencing rage. Valium made him calm and dulled his pain and hatred. I was able to show him that I could tolerate his rage by interpreting his action in a calm, serious way and he slowly found words rather than actions to express it. The drug use had begun during a vacation break,

and instead of expressing his anger at me for leaving him Joe hurt
himself. He had been in treatment long enough to know that this dangerous, self-destructive behavior would worry me, thereby causing me
to feel as he did when I was away. Such tit-for-tat behavior is not unusual
and must be explained to patients who are more used to acting than
speaking.

Patients who have grown up with psychotic, alcoholic, or pathologically narcissistic caretakers usually need to protect themselves
from remembering their painful childhood. Instead they seem doomed
to repetition. Denial, identification with the aggressor, projection, and
projective identification are defenses that are hard to give up. Preserving the parental object, which has become introjected, becomes
a life quest. People who have been poorly treated as children often
end up trying to duplicate the past by choosing objects like the abusive parent. The reasons are complicated and multidetermined; one
is the wish for a better outcome, and another is the need to hold on
to the abuser. True individuation has never been achieved, and separations are extremely difficult for this reason. Relationships are sadomasochistic and the cycle of pain continues. In therapy the patient
will try to seduce the therapist into repeating the past in myriad and
often subtle ways. Rather than feel or experience her own rage the
patient often tries to project it onto the therapist. This tendency must
be pointed out consistently over many years of work. The therapist
often becomes discouraged, angry, frustrated, frightened, and sometimes either consciously or unconsciously arranges to end the treatment. This happened with Dr. L. and Miss Simon in Chapter 6.

Leonard Shengold (1989) says in his book *Soul Murder: The Effects
of Childhood Abuse and Deprivation*:

Those who have been subjected to attempts at soul murder require
one quality from the therapist or analyst above all others: patience. It
is not hard to understand why change must be slow: there is so much
distrust. The emotional connecting necessary for insight is initially more
than soul-murdered people can bear. They learned as children that to
be emotionally open, to want something passionately, was the begin-

ning of frustrating torment. . . . [These patients] have been abused and neglected and have learned a lesson: If you cannot trust mother and father, whom can you trust? So a really meaningful alliance with the analyst takes a long time to develop. . . . To accept the analyst as a separate person and then as a predominantly benevolent one takes years of seemingly endless repetition and testing. One must never assume that the analyst will be felt by the patient as working for the patient's welfare; even with the "average expectable" patient, these anticipations of benevolence are at best intermittent. The analyst and the patient must be able to last it out. Given enough time, the near delusion that only the worst is to be expected, sometimes initially unconscious, can be modified by the reliability of the analytic situation: a time and place that can be counted on, the dependable, continuing presence of a generally accepting, nonpunitive parental figure, the persistent attempt to empathize and understand. . . . Interpreting aggression toward the analyst in such a way that the patient can make use of it requires great skill, perseverance, and (again) patience. [pp. 311–317]

Dr. Shengold's last sentence is the key to working with severely troubled patients. Many of these patients have buried and/or split off their rage, and can function quite well in many areas, but the avoided and acted-out rage takes a toll, particularly in the area of relationships. Carrying rage is like carrying a time bomb; closeness and intimacy feel dangerous and are not ordinarily risked. In order to resume development such a person must be helped to recognize, tolerate, and understand her rage in treatment. Such tolerance and understanding lead to acceptance and to the realization that rage is one of many emotions. This happens slowly and painfully through reliving the past with the analyst as transference and new object. When rage gradually becomes object-directed anger, growth has taken place. When the patient can feel both love and hate without fearing retaliation or merger, mature relationships become possible.

Patients need to test the therapist's ability to tolerate their rage over long periods of time. What is really being resisted is the idea of separateness. Severely troubled patients often do not feel differentiated from the object. This may be seen as a developmental arrest or as defensive regression to an undifferentiated state. In such cases the expression of anger threatens the patient with annihilation, fragmentation, loss of self, loss of the object, or loss of love. In order to pass these tests the therapist must remain consistent, calm, firm, and consciously alert to signs of the patient's rage. Signals of the patient's split-off or suppressed rage include:

Missing appointments (especially with no telephone call);
Forgetting to pay the bill;
Coming late repeatedly;
Expressing anger at people outside of therapy (especially on the way to therapy);
Wanting to quit therapy or cut down sessions;
Experiencing depersonalization or even dissociation;
Reporting violent and sadistic dreams that are disavowed or disowned;
Experiences of psychosomatic pain;
Self-mutilation and self-injury (accident-proneness).

Therapeutic attitudes that tell the patient that it is not safe to feel rage are:

Agreeing with the patient's wish to cut down or end treatment prematurely;
Rearranging appointments frequently at the patient's request;
Answering questions before exploring them;
Letting the patient run up a bill or not charging for missed sessions;
Changing policies in general, such as extending session time;
Forgetting or being late for sessions;
Treating the patient as if she does in fact have a time bomb (tiptoeing).

I will focus on several patients in this chapter on rage. All of them had mothers who were periodically psychotic, alcoholic, or depressed and unavailable, thereby affecting their ability to see and treat the child as a separate individual. The patients functioned on different levels. All of them used drugs at different times and turned their rage against themselves. All were involved in sadomasochistic relationships and tried to relate to the therapist in this manner.

Treatment enabled them to recognize and to direct their anger towards others. Permitting these patients to express their rage in the treatment situation with and towards the therapist is a goal that is met with varying success and takes many, many years of analytic work.

Rage is dealt with in complex ways including controlling and distancing others. Distancing protects the object from destruction and merger. Controlling the object denies it a separate existence. Very often the object "behaves" so as to avoid the patient's rage. The therapist is put in a difficult and frightening position with this kind of patient. If she understands that beneath the rage is a fear of helplessness and despair she is better prepared to tolerate and analyze this powerful affect. Also, many patients feel their rage is powerful, and this sense of power is not easily relinquished. When the rage starts in the omnipotent phase of development any appeals to rationality are ineffective. The patient must experience the rage in therapy to believe that it will not kill the therapist. Sometimes the therapist buys into the patient's fantasy/belief system and becomes frightened. When this occurs, treatment comes to a standstill. When treating patients who are very disturbed the therapist will find supervision or consultation enormously helpful.

The first example illustrates the therapist's wish not to "make waves."

Dr. O. came for supervision on a patient she had been seeing in analysis for six years. The patient had recently returned from a vacation that had not coincided with Dr. O.'s vacation for the first time. When Dr. O. handed her patient the bill that included the missed week of sessions the patient remarked that Dr. O. must have made an error. The bill seemed very high considering the break in treatment. Dr. O. said there was no mistake. She told the patient that over the six years of analysis she had always charged the patient for missed sessions. The patient admitted that he had never really looked carefully at the bill and had just paid the amount stated. In fact, the patient had told his friend that he would not be charged for his missed sessions. The friend said, "You really have a deal. My therapist always charges me if I miss any appointments." Dr. O. offered to make up two of the four missed sessions but immediately realized she had made a mistake. The mistake was based on feeling sorry for her patient, but on further reflection she realized that it was the patient's anger she wished to avoid. She rationalized at first that her patient would be narcissistically wounded by a cold attitude from her. Her rationalization, we came to see, was based on a realistic view of this patient, but it is not the therapist's job to protect the patient from frustration or anger. Also, it is important to remember that charging for missed sessions along with any other analytic stance or policy is not meant as cold or unfeeling. The therapist's ability to be consistent is, in fact, a caring attitude.

Psychoanalytic work is based on analyzing, understanding, and being tolerant of the patient's feelings. Any movement away from this stance subtly tells the patient that some feelings, particularly the angry ones, are not welcome in the treatment. Small errors such as this add up unless analyzed by the therapist. The patient's test is: Can you stick to your policies, survive my anger, and still like me? The test often continues for many years and, if successfully passed, the patient gradually comes to see that patient and therapist are indeed separate. The patient's association to telling his friend and sharing the response with his therapist was the clue in this vignette. He was saying, "Can you stick to your policy as my friend's therapist does?" When Dr. O. explored his countertransference and analyzed the enactment with the patient the treatment deepened.

Before and during my psychoanalytic training my caseload consisted primarily of adults who had been abused or severely neglected in their formative years. I worked at a clinic, funded by the federal, state, and city governments, where people with drug-related problems were treated free of charge. I learned a great deal from my patients whom I was allowed to see for long-term treatment once or twice a week.

The first myth to be shattered was that a patient has to pay in order to benefit from therapy. The second had to do with the belief that a patient has to be abstinent (drug-free) in order to benefit from treatment. The clinic's philosophy was that drug use was a symptom and no one was ever turned away for using drugs. Many therapists will not treat patients who are abusing drugs but it has been my experience that the drug use serves as a defense against closeness, separation, and rage. The drug is always available. The therapist is not. It can also be seen as a test to determine if the therapist can tolerate the patient. Adaptively speaking, drugs give the user a sense of mastery over feelings of powerlessness. I have worked with varying degrees of success with people who began treatment while using drugs. (I have not had success with cocaine addicts although I have worked well with people who used cocaine in a limited way.)

At the clinic I worked with people of various nationalities, religions, socioeconomic levels, and genders. People came of their own free will, because of the court system, or as a requirement of the welfare system. Some came with motivation to change, others developed motivation to change, some stayed just to fulfill a requirement, and some dropped out. All of the people who stayed in treatment eventually became aware of the intense rage that they buried—some by using drugs (heroin and marijuana were favored in those days), others by employing other defenses. Some were criminals, some were college students or graduates, some held jobs, and some were on welfare. There were transvestites, transsexuals, lawyers, teachers, exhibitionists, prostitutes, medical doctors, business people, housewives, artists, thieves, athletes, actors, and I'm sure others I've forgotten. I saw most of my patients in individual psychotherapy for 50-minute sessions, once or twice a week. I also led groups.

Many of the therapists at the clinic practiced gestalt therapy and their patients vented anger and rage on the pillows and dummies they used. I was in psychoanalytic training, so words were my medium. Of course much acting out went on, but being listened to in a nonjudgmental way on a regular basis over a long period of time enhanced the value of words to these people. Patients would give up drug use eventually and sometimes they would have relapses. Others continued using for long periods of time. Sometimes they overdosed and died. Some used methadone but no matter what they did, they had a place to come to try to use words to express themselves, a place that accepted them as they were. In *The Analysis of the Self*, Heinz Kohut (1972) talked about the analyst as a replacement for drugs. This seemed to hold true in many cases. In other cases the drug use seemed to be based on anger and despair. Once the therapist was seen as genuinely curious and nonjudgmental the patient often acknowledged these feelings. I never met a drug abuser who beneath the braggadocio did not feel frightened and alone.

The patient I want to focus on in this chapter is not from the clinic but she might well have been. I came to know her through a supervisee with whom I worked for eight years. This supervisory experience was difficult and rewarding: difficult because the patient was in so much pain, and rewarding because the student was so talented and valiant. All three of us: Ms. C. (the student), Mrs. Skye (the patient), and I grew in immeasurable and permanent ways.

Ms. C. is a social worker with analytic training. She works part time at a mental health clinic and has a part-time private practice. The patient Ms. C. and I focused on in our eight years of supervisory work, Mrs. Skye, began treatment when she was 35. She initially went to Ms. C. for marriage counseling with her husband. This lasted for only a few months because her husband would not continue. The couple eventually divorced, with Mrs. Skye receiving custody of their 3-year-old son.

Mrs. Skye started abusing alcohol at age 11 and heroin at 15. When she finished college she married a heroin user but stopped using heroin with the help of Narcotics Anonymous when she became pregnant.

The younger of two, Mrs. Skye had a brother two and a half years older who was seriously disturbed. Her mother was diagnosed as manic-depressive and was thought by Ms. C. to be catatonic on and off throughout Mrs. Skye's childhood and adolescence. Medication alleviated her mother's condition when Mrs. Skye was grown up but she still required hospitalization from time to time. Mrs. Skye's mother was from an upper-middle-class home, where she had been dominated by her mother. She suffered her first breakdown at age 20 and was hospitalized periodically throughout Mrs. Skye's childhood.

In order to get away from her own domineering mother Mrs. Skye's mother married an airline pilot who turned out to be alcoholic. Mrs. Skye remembers her father as handsome and drunk. Mrs. Skye's father and mother separated eventually and he was killed in an auto accident when she was 10.

Between the ages of 12 and 15 Mrs. Skye was sexually abused by her stepfather while her mother sat passively by watching television in the same room. Mrs. Skye remembers being starved for affection and permitting the sexual fondling while at the same time feeling embarrassed, disgusted, angry, and guilty.

I have given this brief history to explain the roots of this patient's intense rage. Mrs. Skye's ability to finish college and to complete graduate school to become a highly skilled professional with an impressive career testifies to her resilience, something that must never be underestimated. Her resilience was astounding but her self-destructive wishes and actions were life-threatening and damaging to her young son.

When she began treatment she was attending Narcotics Anonymous meetings, working full time (with flexible hours), and raising a son.

Mrs. Skye began seeing her therapist weekly. For the first two years she expressed rage and frustration about her son and husband, her job, and her addict boyfriend. Ms. C. listened and from time to time told her patient that weekly sessions were not enough and were making things even harder. At times, when Mrs. Skye felt particularly overwhelmed she accepted the therapist's offer to see her more often but not on a regular basis.

Mrs. Skye's son Bill began wetting his bed at age 7 and he began therapy at Ms. C.'s recommendation. Mrs. Skye used this for some time as a reason for not increasing sessions. As the treatment deepened Mrs. Skye acknowledged her seductive behavior with her son and her role in the bedwetting. Overstimulation is a cause of enuresis and as she became aware of her need to sexualize closeness she became able to control this need. The bedwetting became sporadic and finally stopped.

The first year and a half of treatment was spent by Mrs. Skye telling about her past and by berating herself:

> *Patient:* [screaming] I'm so base and nasty. A piece of shit. Disgusting, rotten. Why is Bill wetting his bed? I'm an awful mother—my child needs therapy. My husband is no good—he doesn't feed Bill decent meals and he lets Bill get away with watching TV when they're together. Doesn't care about helping him with homework. [This is the way Mrs. Skye grew up.] I have to work and I'm tired when I get home. I have to get up in the middle of the night to change the sheets. I never get enough sleep. How can therapy help? I'm horrible. My life is horrible. No one is doing their job. Even Bill's therapist doesn't help.
>
> *Therapist:* You're feeling so frustrated and angry and therapy doesn't seem to help. Have you considered coming more often?
>
> *Patient:* I can't afford it. It's that simple.

This vignette gives a snapshot of the work for the first year and a half. Ms. C. sat and listened to her patient berate herself and those around her. The constant complaints and bitter, sarcastic, hateful way of relating were difficult for Ms. C. but she persevered. At times Ms. C. said something like, "You're letting me feel just how hopeless and frustrated you are, and you may fear that coming more often would be too upsetting to me."

In reviewing the work we did, Ms. C. and I could not find a definite turning point or event that changed Mrs. Skye's mind about increasing sessions. We feel that Ms. C. proved her steadiness by remaining calm and by not changing the frame. She did not offer to lower her fee because the fee was very reasonable. She did not push Mrs. Skye or offer advice. She listened. One day Mrs. Skye said she wanted to try increasing her sessions to twice a week. A time was arranged and she began. It is important to note that Ms. C. did not specify twice-a-week because she knew that this would not be enough. So when Mrs. Skye increased her sessions to twice, Ms. C. was already thinking about more frequent sessions. (By the fifth year of therapy Mrs. Skye was coming three times a week.)

Here is an excerpt from the fourth year of treatment before a four-week summer vacation.

> *Patient:* I'm so angry that Bill is going to camp. This is the first time he'll be without me—and I'll be alone. It makes me feel so inadequate. My mother tried to raise me and look what she got. I never found someone to go on vacation with. I need to have someone care about me and not a therapist! I'm incapable of laughter—imagine someone spending time with me on vacation. I'm no different out there than I am in here. I'm glad that Bill can get to see that others can be joyful. I do the best I can but I'm a shell—struggling and miserable. Nobody cares to go anywhere with me. I'm sick and disgusting.
>
> *Therapist:* Bill's going to camp doesn't mean he doesn't want to be with you, and my going on vacation doesn't mean I don't want to see you.
>
> *Patient:* He has no chance. He was born into a sick family. Are you telling me I'm a sick bitch for missing my son?
>
> *Therapist:* You feel you're sick for missing your son. We have to understand why, because missing people is natural—not sick.
>
> *Patient:* Does it surprise you that I think I'm sick?

This is one of the first examples of an interchange between patient and therapist. Before this Mrs. Skye seemed to ignore Ms. C.'s comments by not responding directly. Asking the therapist questions meant a beginning recognition of the therapist as a separate person. Here it was done sarcastically and was the first time Mrs. Skye allowed herself to express anger to Ms. C. directly.

At the end of the fourth year Mrs. Skye agreed to begin three times a week after the summer break. These vignettes precede the vacation.

Patient: My mother is applying for disability insurance and she keeps sabotaging herself. All her life she's been crazy. I used to think it was nice when she made fruitcakes at Christmas but now I see she was just obsessed. She couldn't stop. The house was filled with fruitcake. Then they'd take her to the hospital and I was left with my brother.

Therapist: You were exposed to too much too early in your life.

Patient: [sarcastic, loud, tension-filled voice that escalates] Isn't that a fucking shame. I'm sick of worrying about her ass. She's a stupid, pathetic woman. I want to tell her she's an asshole. I try to give her self-respect by letting her manage herself—but look what happens. What am I supposed to do with these feelings? She's an infant, a moron, a retard, and she uses me. If I hadn't been visiting her this wouldn't have happened. I'd like to get rid of her. She's been a burden all of her life. These feelings are killing me. I can't live with Ben [boyfriend] and I can't live without him. He's using methadone and I'm tempted to take some. And you want me to come here more often in September. You're not helping me.

Therapist: You're furious at everyone and at me for going on vacation.

Patient: [screaming] This is not about you. I've come here and I'm falling apart. You're not helping me. Make these feelings go away! I can't live like this. I want to quit therapy.

In the next session:

Patient: I'm sorry for yelling at you. I don't want to be that kind of person. I don't want to be an angry person who has nothing inside except rage and hell. I'm like a burnt-out house, charred and falling apart.

Therapist: A burnt out house can be rebuilt. Talking about these feelings, as painful as it is, is a first step.

When I met with Ms. C. to review this case, Mrs. Skye was in her fourteenth year of therapy. Ms. C. brought me up to date. Mrs. Skye's rage had gradually abated. We saw her need to express it for five years as multidetermined. First of all, she had been dulling it for many years by using alcohol and heroin. The neglect, overstimulation, and abuse she experienced as a child were enraging. The feelings had to come out. The fire had to run its course. As much as Mrs. Skye hated her mother it took many years to let her go by gradually giving up the identification with her. This is the crux of the treatment with a patient who has a psychotic mother. Mother is internalized in order to keep the attachment. Mrs. Skye chose objects in her life that were like mother. Her boyfriend and her husband were replicas of the inadequate mother. Ms. C. was initially seen as depriving and inadequate, too. As she proved her trustworthiness and reliability the picture slowly changed. Ms. C. was identified with and internalized and Mother became increasingly less important. After Mrs. Skye described herself as a burnt-out house she began to relate to Ms. C. in a different way. Homosexual feelings and fantasies were experienced and articulated. Mrs. Skye knew she wasn't gay and she was bewildered by her thoughts. Ms. C. interpreted these fantasies and feelings as wishes to be close. By sexualizing these feelings she could still keep a distance in therapy. Mrs. Skye wondered how anyone (Ms. C.) would want to feel close to her. As Mrs. Skye worked these fears through in the transference she gradually began to see herself differently. She made new friends and began taking nice trips with and without her son. She reported that she had stopped cutting herself, and when she felt panicked she called her therapist on the phone. The self-cutting had been reported in the third year of treatment. Ms. C. calmly asked Mrs. Skye to tell her about it, and the patient explained that she did it when she felt lonely, empty, and deadened. This usually happened before she went to see her mother. The self-cutting in this case had to do with feeling and not feeling. She was frightened of being like her catatonic mother, on the one hand, and of feeling the pain of abandonment on the other. Cutting herself was a way of transferring the pain of abandonment from the inside to the outside. It was also a cry for help. Wearing a bandage was a way of signaling for attention. Ms. C. and Mrs. Skye grew to understand the defensive nature of the cutting. Verbalizing the loneliness and fear of feeling dead and drifting away like her mother did helped Mrs. Skye stop the activity. She could talk about feeling like cutting herself but could refrain from doing it. This was similar to her thoughts about heroin. Mrs. Skye said she would always like the memory of heroin but would never use it again. When she began to enjoy activities like skiing she became accident-prone. Twice she broke her leg and once her wrist. Ms. C. saw the accidents as multidetermined. Skiing trips meant separation from therapy. These trips evoked Mrs. Skye's anger at Ms. C. Hurting herself was a way of hurting Ms. C. Also, Mrs. Skye was afforded good care and attention at these times.

Ms. C. saw the light at the end of the tunnel for the first time in a session in the fourteenth year of work.

Patient: I think something really solidified today. I was sitting with Bill [son] helping him with his chemistry homework—for two hours. Two hours and I didn't get crazy with frustration. I could watch him struggle and I could wait and it felt like we were separate people. With the math I couldn't help so I hired a tutor. I don't have to know everything. It feels so good to let people be. With Ben [boyfriend] I can see him burying himself. And it's not me. I feel bad for him and I worry but I'm not so attached to him. It's sadder in a way but it's realer, too. Seeing that people are not me is like a miracle.

Therapist: It may feel like a miracle but it's because of the years of hard work you've let yourself do.

Patient: We did the work together.

Dr. Z. came for consultation on a patient who had been in treatment for five years. Mrs. Roth had been in three-times-a-week analysis but had cut down to one session a week after four years. The request to cut down is often one of the major tests. The patient is unconsciously saying, "I know you can't stand me; I know you are frightened of me; I know you are disgusted by me; I know you are bored and dislike me; I know you will give up on me as others always have; I don't feel strong enough and I don't think you're strong enough to tolerate what's about to come up; I must protect us from my strong wishes to merge or to murder; I can't afford to let you close because I can't risk trusting you." At such times I have heard therapists support the patient's request, citing respect for autonomy, reality, or resistance. They miss out on the underlying message or challenge: "Prove that you understand me and care about me and are not afraid." This is the most difficult test of all because, in all honesty, at such times the therapist often feels discouraged, exhausted, and angry. The patient has indeed succeeded to some degree in arousing the analyst's fear, hatred, boredom, sense of helplessness, and hopelessness. It is only by facing our own feelings, the induced countertransference and the countertransference based on our own conflicts, that we have a chance to avoid a potential stalemate. Most of the time, once a patient coerces the therapist into accepting diminishing the frequency of sessions she is on the way out the door. Patients can choose to stop treatment without the approval of the therapist and in such cases often resume treatment (see Mrs. Quincy later in this chapter). In such cases the therapist can say something like, "I think we have more work to do and if and when you feel ready I will be here."

The patient's test can happen anytime during the course of a treatment. If a patient does cut down or decides to quit, the therapist must continue to analyze. When a patient tells the therapist that this is the last session I recommend telling the patient something like, "I understand that you are determined to leave but should you think things over and feel like talking more about it I will be here for your next session." If I have specific material, such as anger about the vacation break, I mention that as a possible cause of the patient's decision.

After hearing some material Dr. Z. and I recognized Mrs. Roth's anger and frustration at the diminished sessions. The material had to do with her partner at work who was not living up to his responsibilities. Dr. Z. was able to use this material by bringing it into the transference and recommending that Mrs. Roth go back to the original schedule. After several months of work the treatment resumed at three times a week and Mrs. Roth vented her anger in camouflaged ways at Dr. Z. for letting her cut down in the first place.

Mrs. Roth grew up with narcissistic, volatile, and controlling parents. She was always expected to toe the line and never felt able to speak up. When she shifted her career plans, giving up her choice of profession for her parents' choice, she had a serious accident that resulted in a broken nose and jaw and required extensive plastic surgery. Dr. Z. and I saw this accident as rage directed against herself. Mrs. Roth was so frightened by her own rage that she split it off and lived vicariously through other angry people. She often identified with the aggressor and behaved in passive-aggressive ways.

After several years of analysis Mrs. Roth increased to four times a week. We felt that she needed to make sure that Dr. Z. was trustworthy and not afraid of the anger that was becoming more conscious. Tests around fee, not charging for missed appointments, and coming late were passed. Dr. Z. proved that he would not cave in to Mrs. Roth's requests and that he could tolerate her displeasure.

One day she described an incident involving her mother expressing rage in public. The mother ranted and raved, swearing and screaming at Mrs. Roth, who tried to calm her down. The anger lasted for days and was in reaction to Mrs. Roth's having accepted an important invitation on Mother's Day. This episode, we conjectured, was not unique. Both of Mrs. Roth's parents were extremely narcissistic and attacked anyone who displeased them.

In treatment, Mrs. Roth wanted a calm, mentor type of relationship with her therapist, but as the treatment deepened signs of anger emerged. Subtle but disparaging remarks and actions began to appear. Dr. Z. became aware of his tendency to placate his patient, for he realized how intense the storms would become. But weathering the storms is the analyst's job. Patients in analysis need to deal with the rage that cripples and inhibits them one way or another, making a fulfilling life impossible. Whole character structures are built around suppressing anger. Infantile rage is felt to be powerful and therefore dangerous. It is also frightening to feel anger at one's parent for fear of losing the internalized object. Such rage is often turned against the self and of course, has serious repercussions. Mrs. Roth expressed her rage through volatile outbursts at her office, where she was feared.

Assisting the patient to bring this rage into the transference is the analyst's job. Technique involved interpretation and letting the patient see that her anger was not feared.

Chapter 6 presents more material that illustrates some of the ways rage is expressed. In this chapter I will present Mrs. Quincy, whose fear of her own rage resulted in dramatic splitting.

Mrs. Quincy came to treatment because her husband was threatening to leave her for another woman. Her symbiotic attachment to him had helped this fragile woman maintain her equilibrium for most of her adult life. Now due to this possible loss she began to panic. During the first several years of twice-a-week sessions Mrs. Quincy related a troubling childhood. Her mother was described as icy, stonelike, critical, and unavailable. The therapist was seen as rigid, unbending, unaccepting, and distant. After almost every vacation break Mrs. Quincy broke or cancelled appointments or threatened to end therapy. The therapist had interpreted this as anger about not being in control. Mrs.Quincy increasingly grew to trust him but with every step forward she took several steps back.

Mrs. Quincy was an artist and had a vivid imagination that fed her talent. The therapist's ability to remain calm and steady was tested time after time. Mrs. Quincy sometimes behaved bizarrely in the office and the therapist would ask her to calm down so that they could understand what was going on. At such times the therapist tried to connect the psychotic-like moments to a precipitating event. Anything that threatened the steadiness of the therapy seemed to set Mrs. Quincy off. A change in appointment times, the therapist's move to a new office, or a cancellation might be the cause of bizarre behavior in the office. Mrs. Quincy would touch the wall and think that someone was behind it. Phobias became intense and a fear of losing her identity was expressed. The behavior was treated calmly and with benevolent curiosity. One effect it had was enabling Mrs. Quincy to depend on others while keeping them at a distance. Husband and therapist became more available at these times. Extra sessions were held along with phone contact between sessions and over weekends. With time Mrs. Quincy calmed down and began to look at the dramatic episodes with curiosity. She had often expressed her fear of not being noticed and this fear was connected by the therapist to her mother's unavailability in childhood. She remembered a time when her beloved dog died and she ran to put her head in her mother's lap for comfort and soothing. Mother was pregnant and Mrs. Quincy remembered a hard place where the lap had been. She ran away in anger, blaming her mother for ignoring her. The degree to which Mrs. Quincy projected her own rage and the degree to which the mother was truly unempathic is impossible to know. What matters is that the patient's perception is received by the therapist nonjudgmentally and with neutral ears. It is important that the therapist not join in with the patient by calling the mother horrible because the mother representation often softens over time. As the patient becomes more comfortable with her own anger the need to project it onto others diminishes. In the fifth year of therapy Mrs. Quincy's mother visited. Mrs. Quincy could not decide if her mother had really changed or if it was her new ability to be more patient, but the visit proved to be enjoyable.

In the third year of treatment Mrs. Quincy informed her therapist, who was in supervision with me, that there was "another person" who took over. This other person had a separate identity. She had a separate bank account and driver's license. She used drugs and was a "bad person" in general.

The introduction of "another person" (and another after that) surprised the therapist. After listening calmly to this startling new information and to Mrs. Quincy's unwillingness to talk more about it, he told Mrs. Quincy that he thought the "other person" represented an aspect of herself that she was at present uncomfortable recognizing. He wondered to Mrs. Quincy if the angry, aggressive, bad feelings were assigned to the "other person" so that Mrs. Quincy would not have to feel them, and he offered to explore with her why these feelings were so upsetting.

As treatment progressed Mrs. Quincy introduced other aspects of herself (at first she called these aspects "other people"). One "other person" introduced a year or so after the first was an appeaser. She was described as rational, forgiving, and competent. The therapist helped Mrs. Quincy see that her "other people" were different facets of herself and that these facets represented mixed feelings that could coexist with each other.

The work with Mrs. Quincy was challenging and at times frightening for the therapist but his ability to stay calm and steady made continuing the work possible. At times the therapist worried. He called me between supervisory sessions and we talked about his fears. This extra contact helped him and seemed to parallel the process of Mrs. Quincy calling him on the phone. He also wondered when his patient exhibited psychotic-like behavior if she would be better treated in the hospital. He asked her what she thought. Making Mrs. Quincy a responsible party in the treatment by including her in treatment decisions enlisted her higher ego functioning and avoided infantilizing her. By sharing his concern with the patient the therapist became a model for rational and caring thought. We wondered if Mrs. Quincy's third "other" was a beginning internalization of the therapist.

Would giving Mrs. Quincy a diagnosis have helped the therapist? We pondered that question and decided that it would not have made a difference in the work. We saw Mrs. Quincy as an extremely talented and intelligent person who feared closeness because of her wishes to merge (to be part of someone) and because of her intense, primitive rage that threatened to erase her needed objects. The need to feel close and feel part of another is appropriate in childhood, and when the child is rejected and treated without warmth and empathy the need does not disappear. The need to feel part of the mother at times, if not responded to, leaves the child in a craving state, a frightened state, and a frustrated state. As an adult the wish to feel close is anxiety-provoking, particularly when aggression is not tamed. Certain defenses such as splitting and projective identification are used and become part of the character armor. When a life situation threatens one's equilibrium (when Mrs. Quincy's husband threatened to leave, or the therapist went on vacation) anxiety becomes overwhelming. In Mrs. Quincy's case she became fragmented and lost her identity from time to time. In therapy before the analyst went away Mrs. Quincy felt out of control and filled with rage. Sometimes she self-medicated, sometimes she pulled herself together by withdrawing or plunging herself into work, sometimes she developed phobias, sometimes she lost herself in fantasy, which she often preferred over reality. Whatever Mrs. Quincy did was the best she could do at that time. The therapist could only stand by and interpret what he thought was going on. He could not take away her anxiety. He could only try to help her understand it. Sharing his views with Mrs. Quincy seemed to help. She tried many times over the course of treatment to change the rules of therapy and when she couldn't she would feel angry. She would miss sessions, leave early, refuse to talk, and once she quit for a month. The therapist was there when she returned. These comings and goings might be seen as belated attempts at rapprochement. Mrs. Quincy remarked when she came back that everything was the same. This seemed very important to her. She learned over time that her rage did not destroy the therapist who remained reliable and constant. The therapist did refer Mrs. Quincy for medication in the second year of treatment when she began to feel fragmented and panicked. She complained about the side effects of the medication, saying that they interfered with her work. She eventually stopped taking the antipsychotic and tranquilizing drugs. One positive sign throughout the work with Mrs. Quincy was her lucidity and maturity over the telephone. During times of intense anxiety she and the therapist talked on the phone between sessions. The therapist was always impressed by her relatedness and appropriateness during these conversations. Interpretations he made in the office were often ignored but Mrs. Quincy remembered them and indicated on the phone that she understood.

In this chapter I have tried to show how different patients handle their rage pathologically and how important the therapist's patience and ability to tolerate the different manifestations of rage are. What I find impressive is how uniquely each patient deals with her rage. This is why diagnostic labels seem so inadequate and stifling to me. The benevolent curiosity shown by the therapist along with the attitude of respect, tolerance, and fortitude is what makes therapy possible and valuable to all parties concerned.

I doubt that rage ever disappears in maltreated individuals, but if it is verbalized and understood the need to distance others diminishes. And, although catharsis is not an analytic goal, expressing rage does seem to help a patient feel accepted, sometimes for the first time.

A patient's rage must be considered as a defense against the wishes for close and loving feelings that proved devastating in her past. Tolerating the patient's feelings of love is just as important as tolerating her rage.

From Psychotherapy to Psychoanalysis— Deep Waters

Before discussing how, when, and why psychotherapy deepens into the most intensive form of treatment, psychoanalysis, it is important to examine the differences between the two and to see if there is in fact a definable, recognizable line of demarcation. Historically, psychotherapy has been viewed as problem- or symptom-centered while psychoanalysis is concerned with the whole person. The goal of psychotherapy was seen as symptom relief and the goal of psychoanalysis was a total reorganization of personality through analysis of character problems. Techniques used in psychotherapy were said to include suggestion, abreaction, clarification, and manipulation while the techniques of psychoanalysis were limited to analysis of the transference and the resistance leading to insight through interpretation. It is recognized more and more that each of these techniques is used in both forms of treatment at different times.

Conservative analysts who maintain that there is a clear difference between psychoanalytic psychotherapy and psychoanalysis and assess a patient's analyzability to determine the appropriate form of treatment have been challenged. Gediman (1991), in an excellent discussion of the transition from psychotherapy to psychoanalysis, states her conviction "that practically speaking analyzability is often, if not always, an emergent phenomenon, dependent on conducting psychoanalytic psychotherapy within the bounds of the basic treatment model" (p. 179). In a panel (1987) on converting psychotherapy to psychoanalysis Merton Gill said, "The question of converting psychotherapy into psychoanalysis should rarely arise in the practice of a psychoanalyst because he should be almost always practicing psychoanalysis" (p. 722). Rothstein (1995) believes that "a trial of analysis is the optimal treatment for most people who seek analysts' help regardless of the presenting manifestations of their difficulties" (p. ix).

I will define analysis as a form of psychotherapy in which the patient is permitted to examine the origins and roots of conflict and fantasy by experiencing them as they come alive in the present with the analyst as transference object. Although this can and does happen in psychotherapy, the frequency of analysis (four to five times a week) allows for a more intense experience and for deeper exploration and understanding. The permission to undergo a regressive transference neurosis is given by the analyst's posture of empathic abstinence, neutrality (not taking sides whenever possible), and benevolent curiosity. I qualify the term "abstinence" with the word "empathic" because analysts have a stereotypical reputation as being emotionally unresponsive and silent. The analyst's position of not gratifying the patient's transference wishes (abstinence) can be explained to the patient in a respectful, empathic manner, thereby enlightening and not injuring the patient. An empathic manner does not preclude the patient's expression of anger and other regressive phenomena, as we will see later in this chapter with Ms. Crosby. Interpretation is the analyst's major intervention in working with the patient but this does not preclude explanation—especially in the beginning of treatment.

Things that interfere with and skew the normal development of the transference neurosis have to do with the analyst ceasing to behave in neutral and nonjudgmental ways. This neutral stance does not make the analyst a blank screen or merely a mirror. Neutrality has more to do with not taking sides and with respecting a patient's autonomy. Everything about the analyst that the patient notices or imagines makes her an object of interest and of transference. The way she looks, the way the office looks, the sound of her voice, the things she chooses to comment on make her a person, however accurate or distorted the perceptions of her become. The tendency to make a new person like an old person is ubiquitous and it is this ability to transfer old feelings onto new experiences that makes analytic work possible. This tendency occurs in psychotherapy but the frequency of analysis and the use of the couch make it easier to stay with and develop transference phenomena. The frequency also permits most patients to become aware of and to explore fantasy.

In an important paper, "Notes on Transference: Universal Phenomenon and Hardest Part of Analysis," Brian Bird (1972) speaks of transference as "a universal mental function which may well be the basis of all human relationships" (p. 267). Bird goes on to propose that transference be considered a major ego function "giving birth to new ideas, and new life to old ones" (p. 267).

When psychotherapy is conducted using the principles listed in Chapter 1, transference will develop automatically. How the transference is used is the major difference between psychotherapy and psychoanalysis. In psychotherapy, often conducted once or twice a week, the patient's transference feelings do not usually reach the crescendo heard in the everyday work of analysis. Also, some disturbed patients are not initially willing and able to experience the analyst as separate enough to absorb or understand object-related interpretations. In analysis the intensity of feeling is allowed to escalate and to go on for longer periods of time because the frequency of sessions permits the patient to tolerate the discomfort involved. Once- or twice-a-week therapy is not usually enough to contain the anxiety caused by intense transference experiences. One reason that some once- or twice-a-week treatments end prematurely is that the transference fantasies are stifled and consciously avoided by the patient and left unexplored by the therapist (see Chapter 4).

In this book I have taken the position that a continuum exists. Psychoanalytic psychotherapy is viewed as a form of treatment that can evolve into the more intensive work of psychoanalysis if the two parties agree to go deeper. The decision is based on the fixity of the patient's problems, on motivation, on trust, and on stamina (from both sides of the couch). How and when the work deepens is an individual matter based on the match between patient and analyst. Each patient–analyst dyad sets the course and travels at its own pace. The analyst stands with broom in hand, sweeping the way clear of obstacles. This is not a very glamorous picture of the analyst's work but one that must be considered. What is important is "not the extent to which we may be able to impart knowledge of [the patient's] life and psyche, but it is the extent to which we can clear the patient's own way to it and give him freedom of access to his own mind" (Searl 1936, p. 487).

If the analyst is convinced that the journey inward is a necessary and viable one it becomes her responsibility to inform the patient and to act as guide and companion. Clearing the way for travel is the analyst/guide's most important job. The other trips she has taken (her own being the most important) prepare her for a rigorous journey. This travel experience teaches her that the ability to stay out of the way requires attention and practice. The analyst's tendency to want a larger and more active role must be fought constantly and regularly. Many actors define a good director as one who brings out the best they have to offer in the particular role they are playing. The analysand plays all roles in her life drama and the analyst, like the good director, lets the best emerge. By "the best" I mean the multileveled aspects of all self and object representations, of all object relationships, of all emotions, of all instincts, and of all agencies of the mind.

Using these analogies I envision psychoanalytic psychotherapy as the first leg of a journey that may or may not continue. Before a patient makes her first appointment there are transference fantasies and fantasies of cure. When a patient comes once or twice a week these fantasies and thoughts about the therapy and the therapist continue. These beginning thoughts can be understood as preliminary exercises that strengthen the muscles and motivation needed for traveling. The beginning phase of psychotherapy can be likened to early skit rehearsals. Whether the work deepens into the full-length drama of psychoanalysis proper depends on both parties. In my experience supervising others and monitoring my own work I keep my eye on the analyst's stamina, perseverance, and conviction, both conscious and unconscious, and the patient's evolving ability to be curious, to trust, and to explore.

If the therapist keeps sweeping away the obstacles the patient will frequently find the trip plausible, possible, and worth taking. Many obstacles and fears have to do with trust. If they are understood as appropriate by the therapist and not judged as enactment resistances meant to frustrate the analyst (Rothstein 1995) these obstacles and fears diminish. Seeing such disinclinations on the patient's part to plunge into analysis immediately purely as resistance puts a pejorative slant on things and can result in a power struggle. Resistance is a natural response to beginning the journey inward. The patient who begins analysis to please the analyst is far more likely to come to a standstill later in treatment. This is one reason that so many analysts seek a personally motivated analysis when their required training analysis is completed. Seeking second and third analyses does not mean that the former treatments were not good enough or even lacking. As people mature the journey inward is taken for different reasons and with different capacities. Also, the difference in match often provides new opportunities for understanding. Sites already visited are seen in new and different ways.

The main point here is that psychoanalytic work is not just like a journey—it *is* a journey. If the therapist stays out of the way and addresses the obstacles that are in the way the work deepens naturally. The recent debate about if, when, and how the analyst uses herself in relating to the patient is interesting and complex. It goes without saying that the analyst uses her own experiences and her own transference feelings to understand and to communicate effectively with the patient. Whether and when she shares her personal experience and reactions with the patient is a subtle question that defies rules because just as each patient is unique, so is each analyst. Two people working together over a long period of time develop their own style of communicating, which falls under the heading of match or fit. If a patient can use the analyst's sharing of a personal communication to deepen her understanding both parties will know it. If the patient responds poorly to the analyst's self-revelation, something is learned. The analyst's intuition and style, along with her sense of the patient, determine if and when she discloses something personal. Some analysts seem most comfortable sharing their personal experience when they feel it would further the work, while other analysts are by nature more private. Different analysts have different styles. One might feel that sharing a personal experience will further the analytic process while another believes the process is furthered without self-disclosure. Metaphors are shared as well as analyzed. Humor unique to the dyad is used. Silences take on different meanings during a course of treatment. Intimacy grows over time regardless of self-disclosure on the analyst's part. Essentially, timing is an important element. As the years go by the therapeutic dyad increases its frame of reference.

Why deepen the work into its most intensive form? In the beginning of this book I said that everyone wants a second chance. Second chances usually require the hard, consistent work of analysis. Most deeply troubled people are not sufficiently aware of the opportunities that analysis offers and that without analysis the chances of structural change and growth are limited. This is a strong statement and one that has not been made clearly and convincingly enough. The psychoanalytic establishment has thus far not been able to convey to the public that analytic work is a viable investment of time and money. The most recent excuse is managed care and its effects. Some analysts speak of the death of the profession. A major purpose of this book is to generate interest and enthusiasm among clinicians in doing in-depth work based on psychoanalytic theory.

For different reasons, at different times, the treatment of psychoanalysis has been reserved for only those people who are considered "neurotic." It is now recognized by many clinicians that analysis is the treatment of choice for the most troubled patient. I am speaking of people who have often been considered not appropriate for analysis by many of the traditional analysts who have been practicing for many years and who teach at the major analytic institutes in the United States. Leo Stone's important paper (1954), "The Widening Scope of Indications for Psychoanalysis," has done a great deal to educate analysts to see that psychoanalysis is appropriate and necessary for a wide variety of people. Phyllis Greenacre (1956) speaks of the long working through process required when there has been early trauma. Hans Loewald (1960) discusses the therapeutic action of analysis with patients who exhibit defective egos. Michael Porder (1990) sees analysis as necessary for the most disturbed patient. Also it has become clear that the perception of analyzability is different in England and South America, where many patients, according to the literature and meetings I have attended, seem to be less structured than the so called "classic neurotic."

My clinical experience as a training and supervising analyst at two institutes has taught me that the more disturbed patient usually can benefit most from intensive psychoanalytic work. Even patients who have psychotic episodes are treatable in analysis. Many sophisticated, seasoned, erudite analysts, both in the past and today, like Edith Jacobson and Sheldon Bach, to name only two, have been analyzing these patients for years but for some reason the traditional, conservative view that analysis is meant only for the "neurotic" seems to prevail.

While writing this book I saw two cases in consultation that fortified my belief that psychoanalytic work is required for deep and lasting change.

A 50-year old woman suffering from major depressive episodes with increasing frequency had been on medication and in therapy for many years. The weekly therapy was called "supportive" and consisted of advice and encouragement. The patient was intelligent and curious about the whys behind her symptoms and fears, and she was aware that her life was not getting any better with the advice her therapist gave. A friend of hers whom I had treated twelve years ago suggested she consult with me. Had this friend not made the suggestion this woman might never have become aware of the opportunity to avail herself of a more in-depth treatment. Her psychopharmacologist did not believe in therapy and her "supportive" therapist seemed content to continue supportive work. I recommended that this woman begin working with a psychoanalyst who could decide with her if analysis would be the treatment of choice.

A 41-year-old man consulted on the advice of his physician. He suffered from a travel phobia and an inability to perform sexually with his fiancée. He had been in therapy for three years—once or twice a week— with an analyst who explained that he was suffering from castration anxiety due to childhood events. The patient found this explanation somewhat interesting but not at all helpful. Intellectual explanations were not what this man needed. Why the analyst did not work with the transference was not clear to me but this was not the first time I had heard of an analyst who worked in this exclusively intellectual way.

I hope that this book, along with the books and articles already written and quoted in earlier chapters, will encourage clinicians to reexamine their practices with an eye to deepening the work towards the analytic end of the continuum, because many patients do best with in-depth work.

How, when, and why does psychotherapy lead to psychoanalysis? I have found that if the initial phase of treatment, sometimes referred to as psychoanalytic psychotherapy or psychotherapy preparatory for psychoanalysis, is conducted with analytic principles and techniques, it can and often does evolve naturally into the form of psychotherapy called psychoanalysis. I have used the idea of deepening the treatment to avoid, when possible, the need to delineate one form of treatment from another. This will offend psychoanalysts who take a purist, more orthodox approach. However, I believe that it is just such an approach that has made the word "psychoanalysis" unpopular and mistrusted by the public. Psychoanalysis is a form of treatment that permits and promotes regression in the service of growth. The use of the couch and the frequency of sessions assist the regression and also make it possible to endure. But the analyst's attitude and the match between patient and analyst are, in my mind, of utmost importance in allowing this to happen. We have all seen that frequency and use of the couch mean relatively little in establishing an atmosphere of safety. It is the analyst's ability to show that going deeper is valuable and that she can be a reliable guide on a journey into the unknown that makes the process plausible and possible for the patient.

With certain exceptions, psychoanalysis has become the treatment of choice for a majority of patients who have crossed my threshold, both in my clinic days and in my private practice. This has also been the case with many of those whom I supervise and with whom I consult. Reasons for this have to do with the fact that severely troubled patients and those with a characterological basis to their difficulties do not respond in deep and lasting ways to less intensive treatment. It takes many years of everyday work for a patient to resume development and deal more appropriately with conflict. The premise of this book is that "wading in" to this intensive work is often necessary for the patient whose issues are framed and permeated by mistrust.

I am saying that the analytic process is required for deep and lasting change; that analyzability depends on the capacity for self-reflection, which can be found in patients across the diagnostic spectrum; and that engaging the patient in a psychoanalytic process often involves a period of testing from both sides of the couch. These tests are subtle, often unconscious, and have to do with the concept of the analyst as a new object, as well as a transference object (Loewald 1960), and with establishing a rapport, a feeling that the two parties can work with each other. Some call this a *match* or a *fit*. Giovacchini (1994), in discussing his therapeutic philosophy, says:

> Rather than relying on the formal elements of the patient's psychopathology, I was more concerned about the interaction between myself and the patient. This shifts the focus of the indications and contraindications for analysis. Treatability depends on the 'fit' between analyst and patient. Some analysts can treat patients that others cannot. I felt much more comfortable when I stopped thinking of rules and tried to adapt myself to what I felt was best for the analytic process. [p. 16]

Very often, and again this cuts across the diagnostic spectrum, a potential analysand needs a slower pace to establish the trust necessary to form an alliance. The idea of putting feelings into words, the freedom to talk about whatever comes to mind, and to be curious about oneself are, by and large, new opportunities leading to new experiences.

Repeating what I said in Chapter 2, diagnosis is not what should determine a patient's ability and need for psychoanalytic treatment. There are so-called "classic neurotics" who are not self-reflective and whose rigidity precludes analytic work, and there are so-called "borderline" patients who do beautifully in analysis because of this capacity. It takes varying amounts of time to assess a patient's capability, and diagnostic labels can hinder and cramp the analyst's ability to make the determination.

Realistically we are not able to do analytic work with every patient. We have limited resources of time, patience, and economic freedom, depending on our individual needs and interests at any given point in our personal and professional lives. With our training and with our intuition we learn to discriminate. We each do best with certain types of patients. In our need to be scientific, however, we sometimes tend to obfuscate personal preference with differential diagnosis. We may even use our education and knowledge to cover our gut feelings (our own resistance), and we rely on intellectual reasons for making the decision to analyze or to offer therapy. Finally, it is important to note that we have not been sufficiently taught that analysis can evolve from psychotherapy.

Things other than diagnosis and resistance that determine the therapist's decision regarding the course a treatment takes are:

Where we are in building a practice;
Where we are in our training;
What our specific interests are at a given time;
Issues we have not worked through in our own analyses that frighten us in certain patients;
Specific problems we are dealing with in our personal lives that resonate or echo too realistically with a patient (illness, death, divorce, etc.);
Our financial situation. Can we reduce our fees when appropriate?;
The conviction with which we feel that analysis is effective. This applies to those clinicians who have not experienced a positive analysis.

When you are trained as both analyst and therapist you find yourself doing both kinds of work. A thorough knowledge of the theory and technique of psychotherapy is invaluable in treating the so-called "widening scope" patients. These patients rarely begin treatment requesting psychoanalysis, and in many cases they require analysis in order to address conflict and resume development. The literature on analyzability is vast and important, but the subject of the analyst's willingness to analyze is just starting to be touched and is equally important.

In his address to the Board on Professional Standards of the American Psychoanalytic Association in December of 1988, Shelly Orgel (1989) said:

Becoming and being a psychoanalyst mobilizes a continuous, at least partly unconscious struggle against the wish not to become a psychoanalyst. Unconscious conflict is a fact of human existence which psychoanalytic treatment unleashes in both analyst and patient but never fully or permanently resolves in either . . . I have seen evidence in students, colleagues, and in myself that defenses against the emergence and exposure of the analyst's terrifying and/or forbidden drives take the form of resistance to doing analysis in much the same way, if less fixedly and intently, as they do to being a patient in psychoanalysis. [p. 532]

Giovacchini (1994) said on this subject:

I have frequently wondered about how willing analysts are to analyze. Most of my patients have seen at least one and more often two to three analysts before me. Their descriptions of previous therapies may have undergone considerable distortion, but there are enough similarities in various histories from which some general conclusions can be drawn. Basically, their former therapists abandoned analysis and sought to be helpful by giving the patient support in handling difficult reality problems. [pp. 16–17]

Technically speaking, this tendency on the therapist's part to be helpful by giving the patient support in handling difficult reality problems seems to me to be the most frequent mistake analysts make. It is a mistake that can be rectified and, if not, it usually heralds the end of treatment. I am not suggesting that the analyst always needs to be silent or to throw a question back to the patient. However, there are so many ways to respect a patient's autonomy while engaging her in a problem-solving way that the error of giving advice must be based not on lack of technical skill but instead on the analyst's countertransference or unresolved conflict.

As we accept that psychotherapy can deepen, and as we become increasingly comfortable in examining our own resistance to doing analytic work, we find that more and more patients are indeed analyzable and require analysis in order to change. This recognition comes at a time when we hope that psychoanalysis will become more acceptable to the public. And, indeed, one may have much to do with the other! Inflexibility has been a profound and pervasive criticism of analysts for the past fifty years. It used to be taught (and still is in some training programs) that therapy would interfere with establishing an analytic process. Many people nowadays come to our offices prepared to undertake once-a-week therapy (sometimes referred to as counseling), and know little about psychoanalytic work. During the consultation phase I have found that mentioning psychoanalysis as a possible option is often helpful. I tell the patient that this in-depth work is most effectively done four or five times a week. I explain that consistency makes the work easier, just as it does in learning any new skill. Depending on the patient I might use an analogy of learning a new language or sport. Many people know nothing about this form of treatment and even if they are not ready to make such a commitment the seed is planted. If and when it grows depends on how patient and analyst pass the tests. For those patients who are ready to make the commitment I suggest that we begin immediately, if we can arrange the time. If a patient is clearly not ready to hear about the commitment involved in psychoanalysis I say that psychoanalytic work is best done from two to five times a week and that as we go along we can decide on the appropriate frequency. This sounds contradictory but clinical judgment and common sense alert us to a patient's need to wade in.

Busch (1995), in discussing the establishment of an analytic frame, says, "While many forms of treatment offer understanding, what is unique about psychoanalysis is that it sets into motion a process that allows for the development of a self-analytic capacity" (p. 466). I have found that phrases such as:

"What do you make of that?"
"What comes to mind about that?"
"How did that feel to you?"
"Can you talk more about that so we can figure it out?"

used in the beginning phase of work encourage the patient's introspective capacity and also inform her that the work is a collaboration.

Busch (1995) also makes the important point that if the analyst alone makes the interpretations "it skews the analytic process in a way that can threaten the analysand's inclusion" (p. 465).

As we know, transference fantasies and fantasies of cure exist even before the initial contact with the therapist is made. As psychoanalytically oriented therapists we are trained to recognize and to use the transference. As analysts we learn to let it develop to its fullest potential, with the end result or goal being the patient's experiencing full emotional resonance rather than partial intellectual insight. We do not act as advisors, teachers, or role models, although patients experience the process as an education, at times a comfort, and will internalize some of our traits and ways of being. Our aim is to listen, to encourage the patient to reflect, to point out connections and what they mean when we feel the time is right. We do this on a regular basis, every working day when possible, establishing a rhythm appropriate to intensive work. When the patient is ready she uses the couch to minimize distractions. We set up conditions of work (fee, schedule, and vacation time) early in treatment, to clear the field for concentration without interruption.

This leads to the process of *working through* versus the *working out* so often done in less analytically informed treatments (Greenacre 1956). Working out is a process utilizing the intellectual awareness of certain ways of behaving, with or without some degree of insight into the roots of the behavior. Dysfunctional patterns are identified and the patient is urged, encouraged, or supported to consciously change old emotional reactions into new ones. Working through is a very different story, although it involves a degree of working out at times. It is what distinguishes psychoanalysis from psychotherapy (although it can occur in limited editions in psychotherapy).

Working through is the everyday understanding and confirmation, on the deepest levels and from different angles, of the roots of behavior and perception via the transference. It is the work that makes insight useful. We have all heard comments like, "So what? Now I know that my mother was depressed. How does knowing that help me now?" Such insight becomes useful if it is arrived at through a conscious experience with the analyst in the present, which then illuminates the past. The family myth may be that mother was depressed, as indeed she may have been, but how that depression was experienced by the patient, and how he or she felt about it and dealt with it, is a unique story that can be revived and reworked in the analysis.

In the everyday work of analysis the patient reexperiences, on an affective level, such feelings as joy, rage, sadness, abandonment, anxiety, shame, guilt, envy, passion, hate, and love with the analyst as transference object.

In my experience the patient comes to realize that, as he or she feels safer and becomes more curious and involved in the process, it becomes logical to increase sessions. If the analyst works five days a week there is no reason to see the patient less frequently. This may entail a fee adjustment and that, of course, is a personal issue. Everyday work makes it easier for both partners to carry over material and affect from session to session. Most of my patients notice the benefit of increasing sessions from three to four times a week and then request the fifth hour.

Ms. Abbot had a repressed fantasy that she had caused the sudden infant death of her 4-month-old brother when she was a little over 2 years old. This fantasy, which emerged slowly in an analysis that began as psychotherapy, aroused mixed feelings of grandiosity, impotence, and remorse that colored her development and affected her life. Because she repeatedly set up situations that fostered her belief in her omnipotent power, it took many years of two-, three-, four-, then five-times-a-week work to see that she could not control people. When she could not control the analyst, she became enraged and then depressed. She was eventually able to mourn her imagined power, which gave her room to experience her real effectiveness at work and in close relationships. She also had to work through her guilt about being a survivor. Greenacre (1956) wrote of the very long working-through process required when reality coincides with a wished-for fantasy. So in Ms. Abbot's case analysis was necessary. Every 2-year-old wishes for the disappearance of a newborn sibling and in Ms. Abbot's case the wish came true. A less intense form of treatment for this intelligent, insight-

ful woman would have proved frustrating because intellectual awareness alone would not have helped.

Mrs. Briggs worked in analysis for several years before we began to
realize that as a child she had enjoyed and even provoked her hysteri-
cal mother's tantrums on some level. During her mother's sometimes
violent outbursts she could feel superior and in control, and could
commiserate as a partner with her father. She tried valiantly and repeatedly to provoke her analyst as she had provoked her mother. When
she failed, and as the meanings of her behavior and fantasies were
worked through in the transference, she became able to face her guilt
and to forgive herself and her mother. She began to see her mother in
a different light. The formerly hidden good aspect of her mother came
into view. Mrs. Briggs's envy evolved to admiration and as she freed
herself from crippling guilt she became able to compete as a woman.
The changes in her way of dressing, her posture and carriage, her tone
of voice, and ways of relating to men all indicated that being a woman
felt safe and satisfying. I don't think this could have been accomplished
in once- or twice-a-week treatment because it was the consistent, intensive work that allowed the transference to reach a crescendo. The
work was difficult, emotionally draining, and eventually rewarding.

Mrs. Briggs's history as a heroin addict would have disqualified her
from most analytic clinics despite her having completed a rehab program. In a seminar I was attending when Mrs. Briggs began treatment,
she was diagnosed as a borderline with narcissistic features and not a
candidate for analysis. I mention this to support my earlier point that
diagnostic categories can be limiting, can cloud the picture, and can
even be harmful if they obscure our view of the possibilities for treatment. Mrs. Briggs's ability to be self-reflective, her intelligence, and her
resilience saw her through a twelve-year analysis.

Dr. A. consulted on Mr. Lopez (see Chapter 3) when she moved
from the clinic to her private practice. Mr. Lopez had come to the
clinic as a condition of his probation for selling drugs on his college
campus. Dr. A. listened to him twice a week for two and a half years
as he told his story of a seductive mother and an ailing father who

died before Mr. Lopez began college. His childhood had been spent distancing himself from his intrusive, often out-of-control mother, and keeping the lid on his building rage. Dr. A. made connections when possible, demonstrated that she could sit with him in silence, explained at times that he feared her intrusion, but mostly she listened. She passed his tests that involved trying to get her to shift from her abstinent, neutral stance. At one point he insisted that she use his first name. Dr. A. chose instead to invite him to explore his wish. Another time he became enraged when Dr. A. explained that bringing coffee to a session was not part of their work and suggested that they understand his behavior. Some analysts may have seen Mr. Lopez as in need of parameters (changes in the analytic frame). One of the growth-promoting aspects of analytic work is establishing boundaries and enlisting the patient's ego in adhering to them. Tactful explanations from the therapist are far more helpful than changing policies. Rigid conformity to rules is certainly not appropriate but a collaborative approach to treatment between patient and therapist lends itself to deepening the work and speaks to the patient at her highest level.

Mr. Lopez began to see that he was testing Dr. A.'s ability to remain calm in the face of his tantrum-like behavior, and as she passed his tests he began to feel safe. One of the most common themes I have come across in doing supervision is the view that such incidents require parameters due to the patient's inability to tolerate frustration. It is the handling of such requests and demands of the patient that can make or break a treatment. The therapist's use of tact in such instances is crucial to maintaining a safe environment and conveying real respect for the patient and the process. I have heard many therapists say that parameters are necessary in such cases. In Mr. Lopez's case, a parameter would have made it difficult to develop the trust he needed to continue the analytic work. He would have seen a parameter as a message that Dr. A. was avoiding his anger.

Mr. Lopez's borderline diagnosis did not help in formulating a treatment plan or in assessing his prognosis. As the years passed, he finished college, got a good job, began dressing appropriately, and made friends. However, his relationships with women remained problematic. After two and a half years of work at the clinic Dr. A. announced that she would be opening a private practice, and told Mr. Lopez that he could decide whether to continue at the clinic with another therapist or to see her privately. His fantasies, fears, anger, and pleasure at "graduating," as he put it, were worked on and explored for several months, and he decided to see Dr. A. in her private practice. Mr. Lopez expressed curiosity about the couch and he began using it as he felt secure and understood its purpose. This freed him to work more deeply with his transference feelings, and he increased his sessions to three and then four times a week.

Analysis had evolved from psychotherapy, perhaps not as smoothly as it sounds, but it did evolve. Mr. Lopez's ability to work with the transference enabled him to proceed with working through on its deepest levels. The shame about his mother's inappropriate behavior surfaced as did the sense of entitlement, rage, and guilt he felt. With the analyst as new object, Mr. Lopez painfully and slowly gave up acting on his sadistic impulses with women and eventually with Dr. A. in the transference, and he became involved in some satisfying relationships.

What made the analysis possible was an increasing ability for self-reflection that developed during the initial phase of psychoanalytic work. During that time Mr. Lopez came to know Dr. A. as a reliable, neutral, nonjudgmental person who was genuinely concerned and attentive. He realized and came to respect that there were no fast answers for him, and he learned to appreciate Dr. A.'s ability to be quiet and let him see where his thoughts led. He saw that she could remain calm in the face of his tantrums, and that she would not be seduced into changing her behavior just because he wanted her to. He learned that she could be flexible when appropriate, and in general he learned that he could trust her. This trust, however, did not preclude or inhibit his transference feelings or fantasies. It did strengthen the working alliance, which was there even when it seemed to disappear. It is not uncommon for the clinician to worry when days or weeks go by with no sign of it except for a nod, maybe a hello or a goodbye. Coming to appointments is an expression of trust and not having to be polite is an expression of freedom. Experience teaches us to wait out the storms, and there were many storms over the years.

Had Mr. Lopez stayed at the clinic with a competent psychotherapist I am sure he would have grown. But I also believe that the growth due to the resumed development he experienced over the many years of intensive working through of his conflicts in the transference gave him the most thorough chance for a full and rich life.

Mr. Lopez's analysis was terminated favorably after nine years of work. Termination is a vast subject. Much has been written on the theory and technique of terminating. My focus here is on the word "favorably." Because each patient is an individual with her own life story and her own unique way of responding and not responding to analysis, I see the issue of when to end analysis as an individual decision made between patient and analyst. In Mr. Lopez's case, and in others, the work could have continued. Analysis is a life-long endeavor. But a major goal for the analyst is seeing to it that the patient can continue the process on her own when necessary. Learning to think analytically is like learning to ride a bike. Once it is mastered sufficiently it is not forgotten.

Aside from people who come requesting analysis, all of my analysands have begun at once or twice a week. By the second to fourth year, they are usually coming three or four times a week, many opting for a fifth session shortly after that. They realize the gain very quickly, and so it becomes everyday work in the literal sense. I must add that the reverse does not hold true. As treatment progresses and gains are made, even when the end is in sight, I do not cut down or taper off. When the patient is at the height of a resistant period, or when the negative transference is intense and the patient insists on decreasing sessions, sometimes jeopardizing a job or threatening to move away, I actively interpret and encourage the patient to put the anger and fear into words. As with all guidelines, there are exceptions because each patient is a unique individual. However, the decision to cut down should be fully explored and analyzed lest it become an enactment. The following excerpt from the seventh year of an analysis that began as psychotherapy, provided by a supervisee, illustrates how a patient in the height of a transference storm threatens to end treatment and how a rapprochement crisis was worked through. Failures in the rapprochement subphase of development come to light during analysis. A mother's unavailability or lack of consistency, her difficulty in fostering the child's autonomy or respecting the child's need to regress at times, her quickness to let the child go, affect each child differently.

The following material is from a patient whose physical and psychological development was complicated by a congenital deformity that delayed her walking until age 2. Between the ages of 3 and 5 her mother became somewhat distracted and unavailable due to her father's illness.

Ms. Crosby spent much of her first year in a partial body cast and her first six weeks in the hospital. The analysis had dealt with this preverbal trauma that had been expressed in affect storms and action. The patient's feelings about her deformed leg had been ignored and avoided until the analysis. Exploring feelings about a real deformity is always painful work and the analytic frame makes it possible. Here the analyst is seen as the mother who could not cure the deformity and who was held responsible for it (this had been established in prior sessions,) and as the mother who was not consistently available.

> *Patient:* [cool, calm tone after a week of anger about the three week summer break] I'm going to transfer to California in February because the company offered me a great deal. I'll have to end here soon to get ready.
>
> *Analyst:* Soon?
>
> *Patient:* Within a month or so. I can make the decision. I don't have to see if you'd let me. I feel that power—it feels good. In the elevator I realized I'm still angry with you. I can end and not have to feel warm and cuddly. I don't know if I want to give up this anger.
>
> *Analyst:* This seems like a solution to you, a way to deal with your anger at me for the vacation.

Patient: You can think that's it. I've wanted to end analysis for ages. And I like being on Prozac. So it's disingenuous to act like I only want to end now when I've been talking about it for a year.

Analyst: I've heard you talk and I don't ignore it. My interpretation is that this is the way you feel today and today you don't like my interpretation.

Patient: It's almost unbearable to be in here with you. My anger at you . . . I don't even want to engage with you. All you want to do is analyze me and you don't know what my feelings are.

Analyst: You have an array of ways to repel what I say to you. It seems you want to spit out what I offer you.

Patient: [Yelling] I'm enraged at you. What's the point of this? My rage is not going away and it's almost unbearable. I really want to strangle you—to do you physical harm.

Analyst: And you're scared of what you feel.

Patient: It's not a good feeling. I want you to do more than just analyze me—and what's the point of this rage? It's an earlier rage, a childhood rage that I've become aware of here and I want to face it better and move beyond it and not be so mad at everyone for feeling so inferior to them.

Analyst: And if you can't do it with me, who can you do it with?

Patient: [shouting] OH SHUT UP! SHUT UP! You had to say that. I come here working on it day after day after fucking day. Oh come on! I was getting to it and you had to prove you're right. [with dripping sarcasm] "And if you can't do it with me who're you gonna do it with!" [pause] It's very hard for me to see you as wanting to help me. Ninety percent of the time I see you as this creep who wants to point out to me what's wrong with me. So understand that I'm hearing things from you in the worst possible way. You know I don't want you to analyze me, I want you to help me. Every time I spill my guts you're in your little chair, looking down at me and I want to kill you. It feels so distant and removed and uncaring. I guess I have to come through this rage and get to the point where I don't blame you anymore for not being or doing what I thought you'd be doing. You're just a person who analyzes. But that's okay—I can solve my problems myself. Like with Fred. I'm not ready to see his weaknesses—his inability to succeed. I don't want to give him up yet. I'm not ready. I still need him. You had to point out that he's not working. Oh, I know I told you but you focused on it. I don't trust you. Are you trying to get me to see what I don't want to see? I don't want to admit I wish he were more successful, more grown up. I don't want to surpass him and I don't want him to surpass me. I'm afraid to bring my anxieties in here because it won't be safe. You'll take it too far. I'm not ready to dump him. I want to explore how I feel and not act. I need to take the disappointment step by step and come out the other side and feel that you did what you were supposed to do and did it pretty successfully. But I'm so angry. I feel like I'm the only one in the world who has ever had to deal with feeling so crummy. You certainly didn't, Dr. Perfect!

This vignette illustrates the intensity of this patient's transference and the working through process. The everyday contact has made it possible for Ms. Crosby to express and to bear her rage, rage that had its roots in childhood when the patient felt inferior and angry because of her deformity. The reference to Fred and his not being successful or grown up stands for the patient's choosing men who do not threaten to leave her and who achieve less than she does. Fred is also a rapprochement figure. At times he stands for the mother and at times roles are reversed and Ms. Crosby behaves as his rapprochement mother. The analysis has worked toward this realization and Ms. Crosby is torn between facing what she has learned and avoiding it by quitting. Years of work prepared the patient to grapple with the realization that she was not truly limited by the deformity. Had she not chosen analysis one can speculate that she would have handled her poor self-esteem and oedipal guilt by settling for less than she deserved and resenting the choice. The rage at the analyst stems from rage at Mother for the deformity and for not being available enough. Because we cannot know what an infant in a body cast is thinking, or how it feels to delay walking, we must listen and watch for clues of preverbal distress. This patient cried through much of her treatment.

She also positioned herself in an unusual manner on the couch, reminiscent of how she lay when in the body cast. The analyst and I surmised that these positions and the crying harked back to very early feelings.

Two weeks later:

Patient: [ten minutes late, rubbing her eyes] All these feelings are coming up. [sigh] Hard to talk about this but I want to talk in a different way than beating myself up. Should I turn down the transfer? Fred called at work just to talk. I was busy so I asked if I could call him back. He said fine but not to forget he was going skiing. So I missed him during the day and thought I would leave a message on his tape. Why do I need to connect with him and reassure him? Fuck it, he doesn't do that for me. Sometimes he does, though, and it feels good. Today I'm anxious about the phone call and analysis. I realized I won't be home before twelve so if he calls he won't get me. I just realized on the way here I feel some of the anxiety I felt about his not being there for me but I turned it into me wanting to be there for him. Like, "Oh, my poor baby." I want to get in touch with him—don't want him to feel abandoned. I want to talk about it here. This tiny instance causes me to get so upset. It reminds me of a time when I was a little girl in Florida. My mom came to find me. I hid from her. She called me a few times and then gave up and went back into the house and I felt like "my poor Mommy"—like I should go looking for her. I wanted her to find me. And I guess that's some of the feeling with Fred. I plan in advance because he doesn't make enough effort to connect with me. But I can't plan ahead—try to be in control. Now I feel guilty and scared, worried I went too far.

Analyst: This reminds me of when your mother was so preoccupied with your father's illness and you felt she was not attuned to you. You kept sending her signals, nonverbally, that all was not right with you. You had skin rashes, hives, and you broke your front tooth, hoping she would realize that you were suffering and needed her. You hoped she would hold you closer, but she didn't. You do that with me by asking for attention and then pushing me away.

Patient: I have several thoughts about that year my father was ill. In Florida I skipped school a lot and the teacher called my mother to say, "Sally's not in school." Another time I rolled around in poison ivy so my mother would pay attention. What was I thinking?

Analyst: Last week you skipped two sessions without calling. You wanted me to know that all was not right with you and you couldn't tell me with words.

Patient: I guess I do have this pervasive sense that you don't care enough. Or that Fred doesn't care enough. He won't come and find me—he lets me drift away. Makes sense about my mom. So what do I do? I feel blue, scared, angry, and afraid of going too far. I can't put feelings in that year in Florida. I carry it all around with me. Someone's going to forget about me. I guess this has to do with the decision about ending. It's the ultimate test of you: Are you going to let me go? But part of me does want to go. It's not *just* a test. I have such mixed feelings. I was thinking how well you listen to me and how you didn't say "Okay, sounds like a good thing." Instead, you say it has to do with you and here. You let me know you're concerned about me. I guess that's what my mother didn't do. She wanted everyone to be fine and have no problems so she never asked questions. I feel like crying. [cries] It's such a relief. If I can play it out with you I won't have to bring it into the relationship with Fred all the time. He's not supposed to be my mommy. I feel like you know what I'm doing. I can act it out here and not put all my needs on Fred. [pause] It's a little bit hard to be here now. I feel shy. It feels intense—like what happened between us was really meaningful.

Analyst: Sounds like this might be the point at which you shove off.

Patient: [laughs] That would be the pattern. What makes it intense is you caring about me. I was right to stay here all these years—to have confidence in you—and you don't go overboard. I don't have you on a pedestal anymore. I think I was doing this massive test and seeing if you would let me go before I was ready. When you said this is the time I would want to get out, that was so right. I felt so anxious, like I want to get out of here. Then I thought maybe I can resolve this and be free of it and not play it out with Fred. I have felt so dogged by this. Always feeling the little girl who feels she has to be reassured, not the woman I am.

This vignette speaks for itself. It shows how oedipal issues intertwine with rapprochement conflicts and it supplies just a glimpse of the intensity that analysis, with its slow pace and frequent meetings, permits. It also illustrates how patient and analyst share the work of interpretation.

In this day and age of fast food, fast money, and quick cures, the idea of long-term treatment is almost jarring. People are not used to waiting, and even in the field of psychoanalytic research there is an interest in shortening the process of analysis. What I find jarring is the notion of a quick or fast cure for a person who comes to my office after decades of living with a certain psychic reality, unconscious fantasy system, and crippling defensive style. What makes the analytic journey feasible is our ability to convey to the patient (and to the public, when possible) the respect, interest, and patience we have for the unconscious. In some hidden corner of every person's mind is the hope of feeling understood and of having new choices. It is the psychoanalyst who is best suited to undertake the journey of understanding—no matter how long or how far. If we keep in mind that our job is to understand and not to cure, the undertaking of that journey becomes possible.

In conclusion, psychoanalytic work is indicated when development has been derailed and when conflict limits one's life choices. The resumption of psychological development and the diminishment of conflict provide second chances.

Being an analyst means choosing a life of daily wonderful, terrifying adventures. Rather than steer for the calm harbors of equilibrium among psychic institutions in peaceful alliance with one's patient companion on the voyage, the psychoanalyst must willingly defy the elemental tendencies of ordinary human nature in order to eschew the rapid healing, premature synthesizing, and the masterful therapeutic activity of which he or she is quite capable. One's pact with one's patient includes a promise to try to live with him or her in continuous conflict, both internal and external, until it is all over—no, even after it is over. [Orgel 1988, p. 531]

References

❖ ❖ ❖

Bernstein, S. (1983). Treatment preparatory to psychoanalysis. *Journal of the American Psychoanalytic Association* 31:363–390.

Bird, B. (1972). Notes on transference: universal phenomenon and hardest part of analysis. *Journal of the American Psychoanalytic Association* 20: 267–301.

Blanck, G., and Blanck, R. (1974). *Ego Psychology: Theory and Practice.* New York: Columbia University Press.

Busch, F. (1995). Beginning a psychoanalytic treatment: establishing an analytic frame. *Journal of the American Psychoanalytic Association* 43:449–468.

Fancher, E., and Hall, J. (1989). *What's in a name?* Paper presented at a meeting of the Society of the New York School for Psychoanalytic Psychotherapy. New York, Fall.

Flarsheim, A. (1972). Treatability. In *Tactics and Techniques in Psychoanalytic Therapy*, ed. P. Giovacchini, pp. 113–131. New York: Jason Aronson.

Freud, A., Nagera, H., and Freud, W. E. (1965). Metapsychological assessment of the adult personality. *Psychoanalytic Study of the Child* 20:9–41. New York: International Universities Press.

Gediman, H. (1991). On the transition from psychotherapy to psychoanalysis with the same analyst. In *Psychoanalytic Reflections on Current Issues*, ed.

H. B. Siegel, L. Barbanel, I. Hirsch, et al., pp. 177–196. New York: New York University Press.

Giovacchini, P. (1972). *Tactics and Techniques in Psychoanalytic Therapy.* New York: Jason Aronson.

——— (1994). An analyst at work: reflections. In *Analysts At Work: Practice, Principles, and Techniques,* ed. J. Reppen, pp. 1–26. Northvale, NJ: Jason Aronson.

Greenacre, P. (1956). Re-evaluation of the process of working through. *International Journal of Psycho-Analysis* 37:439–444.

——— (1970). Notes on the influence and contribution of ego psychology to the practice of psychoanalysis. In *Emotional Growth*, volume 2. New York: International Universities Press.

Grotstein, J. (1994). Random notes on the art and science of psychoanalysis from an analyst at work. In *Analysts At Work: Practice, Principles, and Techniques,* ed. J. Reppen, pp. 27–41. Northvale, NJ: Jason Aronson Inc.

Herbert, J. (1997). The haunted analysis: countertransference enactments and the dead. *Journal of Clinical Psychoanalysis* 6:189–221.

Klauber, J. (1972). Psychoanalytic consultation. In *Tactics and Techniques in Psychoanalytic Therapy,* ed. P. Giovacchini, pp. 99–112. New York: Jason Aronson.

Kohut, H. (1971). *The Analysis of the Self.* New York: International Universities Press.

Levine, H. (1985). Psychotherapy as the initial phase of psychoanalysis. *International Review of Psycho-Analysis* 12:285–297.

Loewald, H. (1960). On the therapeutic action of psychoanalysis. *International Journal of Psycho-Analysis* 41:16–33.

Orgel, S. (1989). Address to the board of professional standards. *Journal of the American Psychoanalytic Association* 37:531–541.

Panel (1987). Conversion of psychotherapy to psychoanalysis, C. P. Fisher, reporter. *Journal of the American Psychoanalytic Association* 35:713–726.

——— (1997). Current conceptions of neutrality and abstinence, G. Makari, reporter. *Journal of the American Psychoanalytic Association* 45:1231–1239.

Porder, M. (1990). On beginning analysis with borderline patients. In *On Beginning an Analysis,* ed. T. Jacobs and A. Rothstein, pp. 163–178. Madison, CT: International Universities Press.

Rothstein, A. (1990). On beginning with a reluctant patient. In *On Beginning An Analysis*, ed. T. Jacobs and A. Rothstein, pp. 153–162. Madison, CT: International Universities Press.

———— (1994). A perspective on doing a consultation and making the recommendation of analysis to a prospective analysand. *Psychoanalytic Quarterly* 63:680–695.

———— (1995). *Psychoanalytic Technique and the Creation of Analytic Patients.* Madison, CT: International Universities Press.

Schafer, R. (1983). *The Analytic Attitude.* New York: Basic Books.

Searl, N. (1936). Some queries on principles of technique. *International Journal of Psycho-Analysis* 17:471–493.

Searles, H. (1965). *Collected Papers on Schizophrenia and Related Subjects.* New York: International Universities Press.

Sharpe, E. (1950). *Collected Papers on Psychoanalysis.* London: Hogarth Press and The Institute of Psychoanalysis.

Shengold, L. (1989). *Soul Murder.* New Haven: Yale University Press.

Stolorow, R. (1990). Converting psychotherapy to psychoanalysis: a critique of the underlying assumptions. *Psychoanalytic Inquiry* 10:119–130.

Stone, L. (1954). The widening scope of indications for psychoanalysis. *Journal of the American Psychoanalytic Association* 2:567–594.

Wallerstein, R. (1983). One psychoanalysis or many? *International Journal of Psycho-Analysis* 69:5–21.

Winnicott, D. W. (1954). Metapsychological and clinical aspects of regression within the psychoanalytic set-up. In *Collected Papers: Through Paediatrics to Psychoanalysis.* New York: Basic Books.

❖ ❖ ❖

Index